The
Vegetarian
Child

The Vegetarian Child

A Complete Guide
for Parents

LUCY MOLL

A Perigee Book

A Perigee Book
Published by The Berkley Publishing Group
200 Madison Avenue
New York, NY 10016

First edition: March 1997

Published simultaneously in Canada.

The Putnam Berkley World Wide Web site address is
http://www.berkley.com/berkley

Library of Congress Cataloging-in-Publication Data

Moll, Lucy.
    The vegetarian child : a complete guide for parents / Lucy Moll.—
    1st ed.
        p.   cm.
    ISBN 0-399-52271-9
    1. Children—Nutrition.   2. Vegetarian children.   I. Title.
RJ206.M746   1997
613.2'62'083—dc20   96-19496
                                                                      CIP

Printed in the United States of America

10   9   8   7   6   5   4   3   2   1

For Laura,
whose Light shines brighter
than the stars

Contents

Appendices

Acknowledgments

Writing a book is never a solitary adventure. An author may feel alone as she stares at the blank screen of her computer monitor. But the fact is that numerous people provide words of wisdom and support throughout the creative process, from the formulation of the idea to the writing and editing of the book.

I wish to thank some dear people who cheered me on while I worked on *The Vegetarian Child*.

My husband, Steve, listened to me as I discussed every conceivable aspect of my book, and he never once appeared bored. He taste-tested all of my recipes, offering straightforward suggestions: "Trash this one." "Let me have seconds of that one." I deeply appreciate your honesty and faithfulness.

My daughter, Laura, served as a living example of the goodness of the vegetarian diet. Some parents have to coerce their children into eating good foods such as vegetables. Laura relishes a plate of green pepper slices, tomato wedges, carrot sticks, broccoli, sweet potato chunks and kidney beans. Just don't ask her to eat onions.

Angela Miller, my literary agent, urged me to do my best work and graciously answered any question I tossed her way. I look forward to our next project.

Suzanne Bober, my editor at Perigee, and her predecessors, Julie Merberg and Hardy Justice, made the writing and editing of this book a joy. They helped shape it into the book I wish I had when my daughter was a baby.

Terry Christofferson compiled the nutritional breakdowns and made a few suggestions to improve the recipes. Thanks, again.

My friends Anne Kramer and Ann Wyant both gave me precious time to devote to this book while my deadline loomed. They invited

Laura to their homes to play with their children so I could write undisturbed.

Edie Rosinski and Katy Kang blessed me with their presence and prayers. Julie Salamonski offered several family recipes for this book—delicious!—as well as heartfelt encouragement. You've been angels to me. Always remember Jeremiah 29:11–13.

I thank Jennifer, Wade, Sue, Gene, Julie, Wendy and Bob for our Sunday evenings together. Each of you has shone light into my life.

Finally, unto the Lamb be all blessing and honor and glory and power and praise. Apart from you, I am nothing.

Introduction: Look Who's Coming to Dinner

A vegetarian diet may be healthful for adults, but isn't it dangerous for children?

This question unnerves every vegetarian parent at some point. It certainly crossed my mind when I decided to feed my baby, Laura, a meatless diet. Family members fed the fire of my worry with their burning questions: "How will she get enough protein?" "Won't she become anemic?" "Didn't you know kids need meat?" Even my ever-loving husband chimed in, "Are you sure you know what you're doing?"

Seven years ago when Laura was born, I had few clues about feeding my daughter. I needed help. A friend directed me to a couple of books on vegetarian kids, but they weren't as helpful as I had hoped. I still felt lost. Fortunately, I had the blessing of vegetarian friends with vegetarian kids, ranging in age from newborn to teens. When I had questions, they shared their experiences and insights with me, bolstering my confidence and cementing my belief that the vegetarian choice was best for both me and my baby.

The vast majority of today's health-minded parents—whether vegetarian, nearly vegetarian or just leaning that way—have few reliable sources for sound dietary advice. Grandma and Grandpa aren't usually helpful, though they want to be; they've been eating meat since they could crawl and still swear by it. Only a handful of dietitians and doctors are knowledgeable about the vegetarian diet for kids. The rest hold tightly to myths, as do some vegetarians.

That's why I wrote this book. In a culture where fast food rules and beef is still king, you need a place to go where you can find support for your vegetarian choice—and get the answers you need.

These pages uphold your decision to feed a vegetarian or a near-vegetarian child with delicious food and a bounty of love. Whether you're struggling with what to eat during pregnancy or how to handle a finicky child, whether you're in a food fight with your family over junking the junk or are trying to understand a teenager who's announced that she's a vegetarian, the questions and answers you'll find in these chapters will speak volumes. You'll get information based on scientific research and receive the collective words of wisdom from parents who've been there.

The chapters start at an appropriate beginning, your pregnancy, and work their way from infancy to the toddler and preschool years all the way to college. Throughout these pages are extra tips and bonus information that underscore the healthfulness of a vegetarian diet for children. Topping off the book are dozens of family-oriented recipes, plus guidelines for planning vegetarian meals and menus.

This is the book I wish I had when I worried about the issues that hound every concerned parent: providing adequate protein, knowing if your child is growing fine, getting nutritious food at day care, handling food questions from relatives, dealing with birthday parties where hot dogs are on the menu. Now I look forward to (gulp!) the peer pressure my daughter will encounter in her school cafeteria and the questions she'll have about her identity: "Who am I? Who do I want to be? A vegetarian?"

If there's one thing I've learned as a mother, it's this: As long as I provide my child with the right ingredients—good food, affection, words of affirmation and a lap upon which to snuggle, to smile, to cry or to just jabber on and on about her world—I've parented well.

And you can too.

As you learn more about your vegetarian child, expect other parents to turn to you as you grow in wisdom. You'll be a beacon of information and insight. Throughout the years, I've fielded more questions than I care to count about feeding children. When people press me for backup data, I could cite a couple of studies, but my best proof is Laura.

She's bright, strong, agile and—dare I admit it—a vegetarian except when she has a hankering for chicken nuggets. When to let children choose to eat meat, especially in a home where one parent is a vegetarian and the other one isn't, is dealt with in these pages too.

With honesty and directness, this book fields the common and not-so-common questions you may have about a healthful vegetarian diet for kids and related issues. Figure on a few surprises as you jump from one section to the next. Count on learning a lot and getting what you want most: support.

Your little one deserves your best.

The
Vegetarian
Child

PART I

The Vegetarian Adventure

1

Just for the Mom-to-Be

You've gotten the good news: You're pregnant! Congratulations. As reality sinks in—and as you religiously keep your prenatal health appointments (please do!), your thoughts turn to food. If you have morning sickness, you wonder what you can keep down. A craving? You or your husband bolts out to the nearest grocery store to buy the delectable of your desires. And as the months march on, you may worry about gaining too much or too little weight. You may even have dreams about wearing your favorite jeans again—after you've lost your baby fat.

As a vegetarian mom-to-be, you may have extra concerns: Am I eating enough calcium? Where do I get my protein? Do I need extra iron or a vitamin B_{12} supplement? Here's more good news: Eating a healthful vegetarian diet almost guarantees a healthy pregnancy and a healthy baby. I say *almost* because even the best-laid plans can go astray. That's the wonder of baby making: the miracle. When you think about how the union of egg and sperm can produce a beautiful baby nine months later, the only possible response is absolute awe.

Eating right is fundamental to your baby's best beginnings. That's why a healthful vegetarian diet is the way to go. Recent studies have shown that even your meat-eating friends are smart to reduce their consumption of animal products. Be sure to check out "The V Diet," page 209, for guidelines for a vital, valid and vegetarian pregnancy.

HEALTHY BEGINNINGS

"I just found out that I'm pregnant. I want the very best for my baby, but I'm biting my nails, wondering if it's wise for me to stay vegetarian. My mom says no. My doctor says yes. Who's right?"

This time your doctor, backed by the American Dietetic Association and the American Academy of Pediatrics, knows best. They endorse a healthful vegetarian diet for pregnant moms, babies and children for good reason. Research suggests that women who eat healthful meals during their pregnancies give birth to bouncing babies in excellent health.

In fact, kids thrive on meatless meals and are less likely than the meat eaters of the diaper set to develop disease later in life as long as they stick with their vegetarian or near-vegetarian habits. Rather than worry, congratulate yourself on snagging a nutritionally aware M.D. Most physicians still have a lot to learn about nutrition.

But before you get too big for your britches—which is inevitable as your baby demands more elbowroom—let's look at the realities of being a vegetarian and pregnant. First, as any dietitian worth her salt will tell you, what you eat is especially important during pregnancy. Wonderfully, a healthful vegetarian diet by definition is just what your baby needs. It is packed with vitamins and minerals, filled with fiber and has an enviable mixture of carbohydrates, protein and fat—and it lacks junk. Admittedly, a vegetarian mom-to-be could gobble up bags of potato chips, wash them down with soda and still call herself a vegetarian. But she is not eating a *healthful* vegetarian diet.

Whether she is pregnant or not, a vegetarian who adheres to a healthful diet selects whole grains over refined varieties whenever possible and eats at least five servings of vegetables and fruits a day. Legumes are a staple, while dairy products and eggs are optional. If a vegetarian skips milk, cheese and eggs, she makes sure to eat a reliable source of vitamin B_{12}, found only in animal foods and fortified products, such as some breakfast cereals and soy milks. She also takes a vitamin D supplement if exposure to sunlight is limited. Her intake of fatty and sugar-laden foods is minimal.

A woman who eats meat, poultry and/or fish can have healthy pregnancies too, but it's best to go easy on nonvegetarian foods. The problems with nonvegetarian foods are many. Topping the list are their high fat content (with few exceptions, such as nonfat yogurt and skim milk), the absence of fiber and the probability of contamination by drug residues, pesticides and pollutants. The fewer animal foods she eats and the more vegetarian dishes she delights in, the greater her chance for a truly healthy pregnancy. Research proves it.

MAKING DIET IMPROVEMENTS

"I'm already in my second trimester and all is well. But having heard so much about the benefits of eating vegetarian cuisine, I want to become a vegetarian now. Is it a good idea to go through with my decision while pregnant?"

You can never start too soon when it comes to better food choices. Both you and your baby will win. However, your question brings up an important consideration: the need to know some vegetarian basics. If you don't know the basics, you might fall into a trap that has claimed many a new vegetarian—substituting eggs and dairy products for the meat that's now off the plate.

Eggs and dairy products are included in the ovo-lacto vegetarian's meal plan, but these foods are secondary to grains, legumes, vegetables and fruits. Your meals ought to be a vegetable bonanza, with animal foods as a complement, not the other way around.

The vegetarian way requires some thought about meal planning before it becomes second nature (and it will). Check out the sample menus on page 147 and try the family-oriented recipes in the second half of this book. They'll ignite a desire to experiment with new foods and new flavorings, such as herbs and spices, which enhance meals without added fat. Develop a repertoire of your favorite recipes, adding additional favorites here and there.

Some people choose to dive into the vegetarian waters headfirst, eating meat one day and banning it from their diets the next. This approach isn't for everyone. Most people prefer a gradual method.

As you learn about vegetarian cooking, you can cut down on meat a little at a time. For instance, you could cut out beef and pork, then chicken and finally fish. Or you might choose to reduce your meat intake in general by dropping one or two meat meals one week, another couple of meat meals the next week and so on, until you are eating vegetarian meals morning, noon and night.

If you still have reservations about becoming a vegetarian while pregnant, keep in mind that health practitioners in general encourage all moms-to-be to make dietary and lifestyle changes. You hear, "Eat a fruit or vegetable containing vitamin C each day," "Have several servings of calcium-rich foods" and "Make every bite count." With a focus on eating right during pregnancy, you have the motivation to make changes. And the sooner you go vegetarian—and learn about meatless meal making *before* your newborn enters the scene and demands your full attention—the greater the likelihood of sticking to healthful eating habits.

SHE'S VEG, HE'S NOT

"My meat-and-potatoes husband, who previously accepted my being a vegetarian, now nags me to pack in the porterhouses, lest our baby be born sick. How can I handle his misguided comments?"

Take a deep breath and count to ten. The last thing you need is a blowup with your husband when you're dealing with the normal emotional ups and downs of pregnancy. Then, in the most loving attitude you can muster, ask your husband about his fears. Listen while he speaks, even though you might have to zip your lips to stop from jumping in with comments. Remember that eating habits die hard. If his mom ate meat during her pregnancy with him, he might believe it's best for you to tuck in a bologna sandwich at lunch and meat loaf at dinner. Even fat-dripping bacon at breakfast might seem nutritious to a meat-and-potatoes enthusiast.

When you believe you understand his objections to a vegetarian diet during pregnancy, address his concerns one by one. If you don't feel confident relaying the health advantages of meat-free eating, get your hands on the American Dietetic Association's position paper on vegetarian diets. It supports the vegetarian way for pregnant and lactating women, babies, children and adults. The reference librarian at your local library can get the paper for you. The citation is "Position of the American Dietetic Association: Vegetarian Diets," *Journal of the American Dietetic Association*, vol. 93, no. 11 (November 1993). Their next position paper on vegetarian diets comes out in 1998. It promises to be at least as supportive as their latest one.

While you educate your husband—and any other relative or friend who doubts the healthfulness of the vegetarian diet—do stick to your decision to eat the best way for you and your baby. You won't regret it.

MORNING SICKNESS

"I feel queasy not only in the morning but on and off all day long. Which foods are easy on my stomach and are nutritious too?"

Morning sickness and pregnancy go hand in hand. That's the unfortunate truth to the estimated 50 to 90 percent of pregnant women—vegetarians too—suffering morning sickness. Some women experience mild nausea in their first trimester only; others have moderate to severe nausea, vomiting, and aversion to odors, bright lights and noise for all nine months.

In every case of morning sickness, apparently brought on by the hormonal changes of pregnancy, your food choices make a difference in your comfort. Miriam Erick, author of *No More Morning Sickness* and a registered dietitian, says that you need to maintain the best nutrition you can despite morning sickness. That means a healthful vegetarian diet, which includes a variety of foods and adequate calories.

If a pregnant woman is unable to take in and keep down the number of calories she needs to maintain her body weight—1,700 to 2,200 calories depending on prepregnancy body size, height and activity level—her body will burn fat then muscle for energy. The burning of fat produces ketones in the body; a high amount of ketones suggests malnutrition in the mother. In addition, ketones may be passed to the fetus and interfere with brain development.

For good health, eat small meals of high-carbohydrate foods and drink lots of fluids. The recommendation of eating crackers and sipping ginger ale seems to have found its way into every book on pregnancy, but the answer need not be so limiting and boring. Ask yourself which categories of foods—salty, bitter/tart/sour, earthy/yeasty, crunchy and bland—appeal to you. Salty includes vegetable soup, cheese and pretzels. If pickles, tea, grapefruit juice or fresh blueberries excite your taste buds, then bitter/tart/sour is your thing. Have a craving for brown rice, spinach, nuts or raisin bread? You'd do well with earthy/yeasty foods. Crunchy encompasses everything from carrot sticks to M&M's to matzo crackers. Bland includes oatmeal, plain bagels and mashed potatoes.

When you know which categories turn you on (or at least don't turn you off), you know the best vegetarian foods for you to eat during your months of morning sickness. Also note which part of the day you are least likely to experience nausea and eat nutritious foods at these times. But if all you can keep down is lemon-lime soda and vanilla wafers, then consume them without guilt. You need the calories and the fluid.

The point is to pay attention to your body and eat what and when you can while keeping good nutrition in mind. During the moments you're overcome with frustration, remember "This, too, shall pass." This truism will help get you through the difficulties of pregnancy as well as the perplexing adventure of parenting in the years to come.

TIRED ALL THE TIME

"I used to be energetic all day long at work and home. Now I drag through the day. Can I make changes in my vegetarian diet to give me a little pep?"

Your body is telling you to slow down because it's expending energy on building a new little person. Be kind to yourself when you're tired and take naps or go to bed earlier than usual whenever possible. That said, you *can* choose foods to add bounce to your step and even enough energy to decorate the nursery. At the very least, you can avoid foods that slow you down.

Start by reducing your consumption of energy-zapping foods or by eating these energy-depleting foods at times when you don't need energy. These include dairy products, which contain tryptophan, a natural sedative; sugar and caffeine (both of which deplete the vitamin B complex that helps combat the symptoms of physical and emotional stress); and any high-carbohydrate food eaten without protein. Carbohydrates, such as fruit and pasta, eaten alone cause the production of serotonin, a substance that has a calming effect—so calming that some people start to nod off.

When you want a pick-me-up, go for energizers:

- ❖ Potassium- and magnesium-rich foods (potatoes, legumes, leafy green vegetables and melons, to name a few)
- ❖ Iron-rich foods (figs, raisins and leafy green vegetables)
- ❖ Vitamin-B-rich foods (brown rice and other whole grains; avoid wheat if your body is sensitive to it)
- ❖ Vitamin-C-containing foods (citrus, melons, tomatoes and potatoes)

All of these foods contain nutrients that if insufficient in your diet can lead to fatigue. Just be sure to eat them with a protein-containing food to head off the production of sleep-inducing serotonin.

Curiously, Finnish researchers found that new vegetarians feel increased vigor and alertness, and less fatigue, compared to veteran vegetarians and people eating a diet of meat and vegetarian foods. The upshot: Eat a healthful vegetarian diet, get rest as needed and take advantage of the times when you have the energy to tackle chores or take a fitness walk.

CRAZY CRAVINGS

"In my first trimester, I turned into a meat monster. Though I rarely eat meat, I had an insatiable craving for greasy hamburgers for three days straight and dragged my husband to every fast-food place in sight. Now I've returned to my near-vegetarian diet. Why did I have such a weird craving in the first place?"

Stories of husbands driving late at night to buy ice cream and pickles for their pregnant wives are legendary. So why not a craving for hamburgers?

It was believed that food cravings during pregnancy signaled the body's physiological need for a specific nutrient. Scientific research, though far from complete, tells another tale. It suggests that many cravings are not physiologically based. That would mean that a vegetarian who craves meat during her pregnancy has no true nutritional need for the protein, iron or other components in meat.

Researchers point to the cultural phenomenon of "pica," the eating of nonfood items, such as clay. Research has shown that pica can't be nutritionally based. Clay, for instance, doesn't provide any nutrients missing from pregnant women's diets. The same is true for food, they contend.

In fact, some psychologists and sociologists believe that cravings are a way for a pregnant woman to involve her spouse and friends in her pregnancy.

While the research continues, scientists agree that only salt and sugar can create a craving because they are the only nutrients that can be tasted. Other nutrients, such as protein and calcium, even if they are deficient in the diet, cannot create cravings because you can't taste them.

In your case, the psychologists might be right. You may have craved burgers as a way to involve your husband in your pregnancy early on. Indulging in a burger once in a while probably won't hurt you, though you may get a stomachache if you're unaccustomed to eating large amounts of saturated fat.

A better strategy is finding a suitable alternative. Suggestions include meaty-tasting options like a veggie burger or a tofu hot dog with your favorite fixin's. Or you could send your husband out for frozen yogurt or a vegetable pizza, light on the cheese. Since your body is in charge of baby construction, you might as well assign your spouse food chores that nourish you.

PUTTING ON THE POUNDS

"My relatives keep bugging me to put on more and more pounds during pregnancy, and they say my low-fat vegetarian meals are interfering with weight gain."

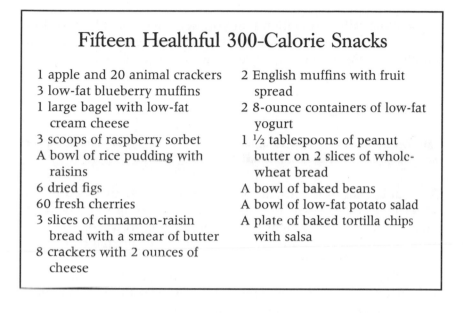

Fifteen Healthful 300-Calorie Snacks

1 apple and 20 animal crackers

3 low-fat blueberry muffins

1 large bagel with low-fat cream cheese

3 scoops of raspberry sorbet

A bowl of rice pudding with raisins

6 dried figs

60 fresh cherries

3 slices of cinnamon-raisin bread with a smear of butter

8 crackers with 2 ounces of cheese

2 English muffins with fruit spread

2 8-ounce containers of low-fat yogurt

1 ½ tablespoons of peanut butter on 2 slices of whole-wheat bread

A bowl of baked beans

A bowl of low-fat potato salad

A plate of baked tortilla chips with salsa

All you need is an extra three hundred calories a day, double that if you're expecting twins. Contrary to the adage that "you're eating for two," it's detrimental to vastly increase your food consumption during pregnancy. Remember, the baby weighs just an ounce at the end of the first trimester and about seven pounds on average at birth.

You'd make a big mistake to overeat. Overeating can lead to an uncomfortable pregnancy and labor. Aim for a weight gain of about thirty pounds, more for women whose prepregnancy weight is low, less for women who are obese. Your doctor or midwife will counsel you on the right weight gain for you.

Spend your extra three hundred calories wisely. The hundred and fifty calories in a handful of potato chips are not equal to the hundred and fifty calories in a large baked potato. The former gives you fat, salt and minimal nutrition; the latter is packed with complex carbohydrates, fiber, potassium, vitamin C and other nutrients. You can also find those extra calories in three large apples, a cup of baked beans or one and a half cups of rice. When you make every bite count, you automatically increase your intake of protein, vitamins, minerals and other nutrients.

Don't buy into the notion that you need to eat more fat. As long as your vegetarian diet serves up adequate calories and is based on a variety of healthful foods, you're doing your baby good.

IRON WORRIES

"My obstetrician has concerns about the amount of iron in my diet and he's urging me to eat meat. Is his bias well founded?"

Meat contains the most absorbable form of iron, an essential nutrient best known for its role in transporting oxygen in the blood. However, some plant foods score high in iron too. You'll absorb 2 to 20 percent of iron from plant foods, compared to 15 to 35 percent of iron in meat.

Truth be told, pregnant vegetarians *and* pregnant women who eat meat need to take an iron supplement to meet the recommended dietary allowance (RDA) for this mineral. The RDA for iron is thirty milligrams. A meat eater would need to eat more than a pound of beef liver, the richest source of iron, every single day to get her thirty milligrams. Ugghh!

The real issue is whether thirty milligrams a day might be excessive. The U.S. Preventive Services Task Force offers food for thought in its report published in the *Journal of the American Medical Association*, noting that "there is currently little evidence from published clinical research to suggest that routine iron supplementation during pregnancy is beneficial in improving clinical outcomes for the mother, fetus or newborn." Moreover, iron supplements can cause constipation, a very unfun problem many pregnant women already endure, and they can interfere with absorption of zinc and copper.

What's a concerned mom-to-be to do? Ask your practitioner his or her opinion, but keep in mind that the practitioner might hold to the myth that vegetarians don't get enough iron in their diets. To allay your practitioner's concerns (and possibly your own), at the beginning of your pregnancy, request a serum ferritin test, which measures the body's iron stores.

If your stores are low, supplement. If not, continue eating iron-rich plant foods with a vitamin C source, whenever possible, because

Iron-Rich Foods

The recommended dietary allowance (RDA) for pregnant women for iron is thirty milligrams (mg.) daily, which is double the amount for adult females aged eleven to fifty who aren't with child. Designed for meat eaters, the RDAs do not take into account vegetarians' better utilization of nutrients. That means you might not need thirty milligrams daily if you skip meat. Talk to a nutritionally aware obstetrician if you have questions.

Here's a rundown of some iron-containing plant foods.

Grains:
1 cup cooked quinoa: 5.3 mg.
⅓ cup (1 ounce) bran cereal:
   4.5 mg.
1 cup cooked cracked wheat:
   2 mg.
1 slice whole-wheat bread:
   0.86 mg.

Legumes:
½ cup cooked black beans:
   3.6 mg.
½ cup cooked lentils:
   3.3 mg.
½ cup cooked kidney beans:
   2.4 mg.
½ cup cooked lima beans:
   2.3 mg.

Vegetables:
1 cup cooked spinach: 4.9 mg.
1 cup cooked Swiss chard:
   4 mg.

1 cup cooked Brussels sprouts:
   1.9 mg.
1 cup cooked beets: 1 mg.

Fruits:
10 dried figs: 4.2 mg.
10 dried prunes: 2.1 mg.
⅔ cup raisins: 2.1 mg.
10 dried apricot halves: 1.7 mg.

Miscellaneous:
¼ cup nori: 5.6 mg.
1 ounce roasted pumpkin
   seeds: 4.2 mg.
1 ounce roasted sesame seeds:
   4.2 mg.
1 tablespoon blackstrap
   molasses: 3.2 mg.

SOURCE: Jean A. T. Pennington, *Food Values of Portions Commonly Used,* 15th ed. (HarperPerennial, 1989).

this vitamin nearly doubles your ability to absorb iron. Have another serum ferritin test halfway through your pregnancy and supplement if need be. Don't be surprised if no iron deficiency shows up. Studies indicate that vegetarians are less likely than meat eaters to be low in iron during their pregnancies.

If you want to skip the blood test and be on the very safe side, take a prenatal supplement that includes iron. It's the recommendation of the American Dietetic Association and the norm for pregnant women in the United States.

CALCIUM CONCERNS

"According to my doctor, I need to eat lots—and I mean lots—of calcium during pregnancy to ensure the health of the fetus and myself. Do I really have to drown myself in milk?"

A bsolutely not. Milk may be the best-known source of calcium, with about 390 milligrams in an eight-ounce glass of skim milk, but it is far from the only—or the most ideal—calcium-containing food. Vegetarian moms-to-be who load up on dairy products to increase their calcium consumption encounter other problems, such as taking in too much protein.

Dairy products are also common allergens, and in some women, milk makes morning sickness even more sickening. In addition, milk contains hormones and drugs that were fed to dairy cows. How these chemicals affect you and your baby remains unclear.

Dairy products come clothed in protein, which might sound like a great combo at first. In the body, however, the protein you eat can inhibit your absorption of calcium. When you're trying to get the recommended twelve hundred milligrams of calcium a day (according to the RDA for pregnant women), you ought not eat more protein than you truly need. The RDA for protein is sixty grams daily for pregnant women. (RDAs are set high on purpose to cover varying nutritional needs. Almost every pregnant woman could eat 30 percent less protein, or about forty-two grams a day, and fulfill her body's needs.)

Because animal foods like milk and cheese tend to be higher in

Calcium-Rich Foods—Minus the Cow

Dairy products aren't the only foods brimming with calcium. Here are some high-calcium plant sources.

1 cup cooked collards: 358 mg.
10 dried figs: 269 mg.
½ cup firm tofu made with calcium salts: 258 mg.
1 cup cooked spinach: 244 mg.
1 cup cooked broccoli: 178 mg.
1 cup cooked okra: 176 mg.
½ cup cooked amaranth: 138 mg.
1 tablespoon blackstrap molasses: 137 mg.

½ cup tempeh: 77 mg.
½ cup cooked great northern beans: 65 mg.
½ cup cooked navy beans: 64 mg.
⅔ cup seedless raisins: 49 mg.
½ cup cooked pinto beans: 45 mg.

SOURCE: Jean A. T. Pennington, *Food Values of Portions Commonly Used*, 15th ed. (HarperPerennial, 1989).

protein than plant foods are, eating calcium-containing plant foods is the ticket to getting enough calcium but not too much protein. In fact, there are many calcium-containing foods that never met a cow.

And here's an illuminating thought: Sunlight increases the body's production of vitamin D, which improves calcium absorption. So lather on the sunscreen, enjoy the weather—even on wintry days, because snow reflects sunlight—and stop fretting over the need to drink gallons of milk. You *can* get ample calcium for the growth of your baby and take it easy on the white stuff.

PROTEIN—HOW MUCH FOR GOOD HEALTH?

Let's settle this question once and for all. Getting enough protein is not—repeat, not—an issue for vegetarians who eat sufficient calories from a variety of foods. That's true for any vegetarian: pregnant, lactating, infant, child, teen or adult.

Study after study has supported the notion that vegetarians receive ample protein. It's no surprise, then, that the conservative American Dietetic Association in its 1988 and 1993 position papers on vegetarian diets has stated that vegetarians get *more* than their share of protein. Even Frances Moore Lappé, who first proposed the theory of protein complementarity in her book *Diet for a Small Planet* some twenty-five years ago, has recanted the need for vegetarians to mix and match foods with different amino acid profiles to attain a "complete" protein.

Nonetheless, getting enough protein is the main worry for new and veteran vegetarians. Just open your mind to the truth: Protein deficiency is not a problem for vegetarians. Truly, with so many wonderfully delicious meatless meals, digging in with a fork and satisfying your protein needs is easy as tofu-pumpkin pie.

Yet the protein complementarity theory has been hard to shake because there is something to it. Plant-based foods are low in at least one of the nine essential amino acids. Amino acids are the building blocks of protein. Essential amino acids must come from the food you eat; your body cannot make them on its own.

But if you eat nothing but legumes, which are low in methionine, for instance, you would not be courting protein deficiency because the level of methionine is high enough to meet your protein requirements. The only foods truly deficient in protein are fruits, sugars and fats. In addition, no one—meat eaters or vegetarians—ought to limit his or her diet to a single food.

Another fault with the old thinking is that it relied on a system called the protein efficiency ratio, in which the egg was considered the "perfect" source of protein. This "perfect" assumption was based on tests done with rats. Though the egg's amino acid profile suits rats to a T, rats and humans differ in many obvious ways, including their nutritional needs.

To find out how much protein you (and not your fellow rodents) need, you may use this simple formula. Divide your weight in pounds by 2.2 to know your weight in kilograms. Then multiply by 0.8. (The multiplier is about one-third higher than most individuals' actual needs to take into account individual differences in the ability to digest protein.) Based on this formula, a 130-pound woman requires 47 grams of protein daily (130 divided by 2.2 equals 59; 59 times 0.8 equals 47.2). The RDA for pregnant and nursing women is ten to fifteen grams higher than for other women. Remember, because this formula is related to the RDA, it is not a minimal requirement.

Excessive protein consumption may translate into osteoporosis (a bone-thinning disease) because protein leaches calcium from the body; kidney stones; gout, and possibly increased blood cholesterol levels.

So the widespread worry over getting enough protein on a vegetarian diet has no basis in fact. Studies show that vegetarians eat more protein than they need. Only people facing starvation or who have a rare metabolic disorder are at risk for protein deficiency. It's time to overturn the too-little-protein myth—finally.

TOO LITTLE VITAMIN B_{12}

"I haven't eaten dairy products or eggs in years. What can I do to calm my fears about my baby getting too little B_{12}?"

Vitamin B_{12}, or cobalamin, is in a class by itself. It is not produced by vegetables or animals. It's made by bacteria. At one time, it was thought that vitamin B_{12} appeared reliably in tempeh (fermented soybean cakes) and miso (soybean paste). However, sanitation practices at U.S. food manufacturing plants have become too clean, so to speak, and the bacterium that makes B_{12} is killed.

Only animal foods can be counted on to deliver B_{12}, because bacteria in the animals' digestive tract produce the vitamin. A dirty carrot or other unwashed vegetable may have some B_{12}, because B_{12}-producing bacteria may be clinging to it. But you won't know for sure, and you'd have to eat *dirty* food. Not appetizing.

A reliable source of vitamin B_{12} is essential to your baby's proper growth. Because your baby cannot get this vitamin from your body stores, you need to provide a continual source through the foods you eat. You can get ample vitamin B_{12} in moderate portions of dairy products and eggs, or you can eat fortified foods, such as some breakfast cereals, soy milks and nutritional yeast. Another possibility: Take a supplement containing B_{12}.

For pregnant and lactating women, the RDA for vitamin B_{12} is four micrograms. Even a single children's Flintstones vitamin exceeds this amount. Don't become overly concerned if you don't take four micrograms every day; the RDAs are guidelines and not minimal requirements.

Including B_{12} in your diet is easy; omitting it can lead to serious and irreversible nerve damage to your baby. When the solution is as simple as a bowlful of fortified breakfast cereal, why take a chance?

FOLIC ACID FEARS

"What's the connection between folic acid and birth defects? I read that scientists have only recently realized the importance of this nutrient."

Folic acid deficiency has been linked to birth defects, specifically neural-tube defects, such as spina bifida and anencephaly. But pregnant vegetarians eating a healthful diet need not furrow a brow. Folic acid, a part of the B complex and needed for the production of healthy red blood cells, is found in legumes, raw green vegetables and whole-grain breads and cereals. These foods are a mainstay of the vegetarian diet but can be lacking in many meat eaters' diets.

The RDA for folic acid is eight hundred micrograms (mcg.) daily for pregnant women. Other adult females need half that amount.

To see how you can meet this requirement, consider these foods that contain folic acid:

1 cup cooked pinto beans: 294 mcg.
1 cup cooked baby lima beans: 273 mcg.
1 cup cooked asparagus: 176 mcg.
½ cup dry-roasted soybean nuts: 176 mcg.
½ cup cooked spinach: 131 mcg.
1 cup cooked broccoli: 108 mcg.

¼ cup toasted wheat germ: 100 mcg.
1 large egg: 32 mcg.
1 cup uncooked strawberries: 26 mcg.
1 ounce cheddar cheese: 5 mcg.

As long as you're eating a healthful vegetarian diet, you will get an adequate amount of folic acid.

PRENATAL VITAMINS

"My doctor says I should pop prenatal vitamins, even though I believe I take in plenty of nutrients every day at mealtime. Do I really need extra nutrition from pills?"

If your nine-month training table packs in nutrients, you probably don't need a prenatal vitamin. Neither does your baby. But taking a supplement won't harm you, and you might ease your mind knowing that you're taking in more than enough nutrients, particularly the harder-to-get variety, such as iron, calcium and vitamin B_{12} (in the case of vegan moms—those who eat no animal products at all). But research has shown that, in general, pregnant vegetarians get plenty of iron and calcium.

Vitamin B_{12} is a different story. Though ovo-lacto and lacto vegetarians receive this vitamin from eggs and dairy products, vegans must be sure to eat fortified foods or take a supplement.

The solution: If you want to be extra careful, take a prenatal vitamin. Just remember, a supplement can't take the place of eating right. A healthful vegetarian (or near-vegetarian) diet comes first.

DEALING WITH WELL-MEANING FRIENDS

"When friends and acquaintances learn that I plan to raise my baby as a vegetarian, I get curious looks and an onslaught of questions. I never know what to say."

Don't pass up this perfect opportunity to educate people about the vegetarian choice. Just tell them with a mix of honesty and gentleness why your choice is the best for you and your child.

Start with health. The American Dietetic Association stands behind the vegetarian diet for babies; vegetarian kids and adults tend to be healthier and live longer than nonvegetarians. Vegetarians get enough protein, calcium, iron and other nutrients for proper health. With the good press about the vegetarian diet, it's not surprising that a 1992 survey by the research firm Yankelovich, Clancy, Shulman, Inc., found that health is the number-one reason people become vegetarians.

Move on to the environment. A vegetarian diet uses substantially less of the earth's resources than a meat-centered diet. It is far less polluting. And it does not lead to the destruction of rain forests to make room for grazing land. These are just a few examples concerning the planet.

State your desire to teach your baby to care for animals. Today's large-scale animal factories are a nightmare. Gently teaching your child that animals sold as food in supermarkets have had a tough life might help her develop empathy for animals.

Surveys show that most people who become vegetarian already know a vegetarian. You're a persuasive example—even if you never speak loudly about your choice. But as long as your friends are asking questions, you might as well trumpet the benefits of the vegetarian choice. When one of them becomes pregnant, she might turn to you for advice on nutrition.

WHAT'S YOUR TYPE?

As numerous as the stars (well, not quite), variations on the vegetarian diet are bright spots of health—as long as they provide variety and sufficient calories. One isn't even vegetarian. How could this be? Let's take a look at the most common types.

Ovo-lacto vegetarian. With *ovo* meaning "egg" and *lacto* meaning "milk," this type includes eggs and dairy products with everything else that comprises a vegetarian diet: grains, legumes (including soy foods), vegetables, fruits, seeds and nuts. It nixes meat, poultry, shellfish and fish. Most vegetarians in the Western world fit this type.

Lacto vegetarian. Eggs are out of the picture (either for health or for spiritual reasons—Hindus, for example, consider an egg a potential life), but everything else is in. That's except for the meat. Most vegetarians worldwide find this type to the liking.

Ovo vegetarian. So long, milk. This type is a variation on the lacto vegetarian theme, but dairy products drop out, either because they cause allergic reactions or because they're seen as by-products of the horrendous veal/calf industry. A minority of vegetarians fall into this group.

Vegan (pronounced "*vee*-gun"). About 4 percent of all adult American vegetarians are vegans, eating no animal products whatsoever. Most vegans also avoid wearing or using animal products, such as leather, fur and wool. Sometimes this type is referred to as "strict vegetarian" or "pure vegetarian."

Macrobiotic. This diet is part of a philosophy of balance in terms of yin and yang. Though the diet may include fish, some macrobiotic adherents choose to omit it and eat the other foods common to this type, including whole grains, legumes, land and sea vegetables, miso (fermented soybean paste), seeds and nuts. Macrobiotics believe food has properties beyond nutrition that affect well-being.

Natural hygiene. This diet, too, has a philosophy behind it. Foods are eaten according to specific food-combining principles to aid digestion. The best-known natural hygienists are Harvey and Marilyn Diamond, who wrote the best-seller *Fit for Life*.

Semivegetarian. Though being semivegetarian is like being a little pregnant—you either are or you aren't—a definition of this type is worth taking a stab at because many people consider themselves in these ranks. Theoretically, anyone who eats a lot of vegetables could consider herself semivegetarian. But more often, semivegetarians, or near-vegetarians, have cut out red meat and/or poultry from their diets or eat nonvegetarian foods infrequently.

Whatever your type, and no matter where you are on the vegetarian path, as long as you eat a healthful diet, you're doing fine. Just pick the one that's best for you and your baby—and enjoy.

2

Your Baby
Birth to 18 Months Old

I n the early months, your baby doesn't seem to need much: a place to sleep, some clothes and a supply of food. But what you give him—especially your unconditional love—is invaluable. Your breast milk, too, is designed just for him. His cries signal his hunger. Be thankful for them. They communicate that he needs you. And as you meet his needs, he learns trust.

As your baby approaches six months old, the fun begins. Out come the high chair and baby spoon and into his mouth goes a bit of mushy food, only to come back at you. Plan on it.

All babies are vegetarian through most of the first year. But you're making the wise choice to keep your child on a vegetarian diet when some of your friends are buying jars of pureed chicken. The truth is, kids don't need meat. Even the conservative American Dietetic Association and American Academy of Pediatrics say so.

In these first eighteen months, you will get a chance to educate your family about the goodness of the vegetarian diet for children. Be gracious as you support your vegetarian choice with science. Your good example would make even Miss Manners proud.

BREAST IS BEST

"Is my breast milk as nutritious as a nonvegetarian mother's breast milk?"

In a word, yes—with one possible but unlikely exception. (See "Vitamin B_{12} and Breast Milk," page 26.)

Mother Nature is amazingly smart and resourceful: Whether you eat nutrient-packed vegetarian meals or a fat- and protein-heavy meat-centered diet (or if you subsist on primarily junk foods), your breast milk will be nutritious. Its mixture of fats, proteins, sugars, nutrients, hormones, enzymes and other substances, including those that protect your baby against illness, is designed with your little one in mind. Your body makes what your baby needs. (One caveat: Moms who are victims of near starvation will be unable to produce adequate breast milk.)

If you don't supply the nutrients in the foods you eat, then your body will take them from your stores. If your calcium intake is inadequate, for example, your body knows to get this mineral from your bones. That's right: It will rob from you, if it must, to ensure the health of your baby.

As the slogan goes, breast *is* best. Not only is it convenient (no bottles to sterilize or infant formulas to mix) and inexpensive, but also it is the best choice for the health of both mother and child. Research suggests that babies who are breast-fed exclusively for six months are less likely than formula-fed babies to have digestive problems, middle-ear infections, respiratory infections, spinal meningitis and certain chronic diseases, such as adult-onset diabetes, immune system disorders, ulcerative colitis and Crohn's disease. Food allergies are also less common in breast-fed babies. Moms who breast-feed have higher stores of iron and are at reduced risk for breast cancer, compared to those who choose infant formula. And those are just a few good reasons to breast-feed.

Experts recommend breast-feeding for no fewer than five to six months, which coincides with the time babies begin to eat solids. But solids won't be a significant source of calories or nutrients for several more months, so be ready to discreetly unbutton your shirt when your baby cries with hunger. When you breast-feed, you provide more than nourishment. You are also showing your care through cuddling, touching and eye contact. This psychological bond between you and your little one has an immeasurable payoff: She learns love.

If you have trouble breast-feeding, turn to your pediatrician, La Leche League, which educates women about breast-feeding (check the white pages of the telephone book or contact a local hospital), or a knowledgeable friend or relative, who can answer your questions and boost your confidence.

And don't forget to nourish yourself. By eating healthful vegetarian meals and sufficient calories, you won't compromise your health as your body produces breast milk. A lactating mom needs five hundred to eight hundred calories over her usual daily caloric needs. Also nourish your spirit by allowing yourself the time and pleasure of breast-feeding. True, middle-of-the-night feedings can tire out the most energetic mom, but it won't be long before your baby is sleeping through the night (at least most of the time).

PESTICIDES AND BREAST MILK

"I wonder about the pesticides and other 'cides' on the vegetables and fruits I eat. Do I pass on these chemicals to my baby?"

When you eat vegetables and fruits that have been sprayed with pesticides, herbicides, fungicides and insecticides, your baby gets a mouthful of these yuckies too. Although the thought of it is enough to spoil your appetite and cause concern for your baby, don't swear off produce. It would be more harmful to scrap all vegetables and fruits, which are rich in all sorts of nutrients including antioxidants, which protect against cancer and other diseases.

A consolation may be knowing that by skipping meat, you're doing your baby a big favor. Animals are "bioaccumulators," meaning that when they eat corn or other crops sprayed with pesticides, the chemicals become stored in their fat. If you feast on a steak or on other meat products, the chemical toxins from the pesticide-treated feed plus any residues from drugs given to the animals enter your body and are stored in your fat too. If you then breast-feed your baby, the heavy load of toxins accumulates in the baby's body. He's a tiny victim of bioaccumulation.

So what's a mother to do?

The best tactic is reducing your baby's exposure to pesticides by eating organic (chemical-free) fruits and vegetables. There are two methods you can choose. The first is foolproof: Grow an organic garden. You'll need good soil, which you can improve with compost or a store-bought, chemical-free fertilizer. Have a plan to reduce produce-munching bugs by planting herbs or flowers that repel insects, adding plant-friendly insects to your garden that lunch on other insects and using nontoxic soaps to kill insects. Check out your library or bookstores for books on organic gardening.

The second method is buying organic produce at farm stands, natural food stores or supermarkets. Look for produce that's certified organically grown so you get what you're paying for. Some states, such as California, have certification, but as of the mid-1990s, there are no federal standards.

When you can't buy organic produce, you can still reduce the pesticides in your diet by peeling or scrubbing vegetables and fruits. With lettuces or other foods that can't be scrubbed or peeled, wash them in a mild dish detergent and rinse well. Unfortunately, careful washing and peeling doesn't always suffice. Some produce, even after proper preparation, may have pesticide residues, according to a report from the U.S. Department of Agriculture's Pesticide Data Program. The report found that 61 percent of six thousand vegetable and fruit samples had measurable residues from at least one pesticide.

Another tactic is to stop buying produce grown outside the United States. U.S. regulations prevent the use of certain dangerous pesticides on American crops, but these pesticides may still appear on foods sold in your neighborhood supermarket. This nasty phenomenon has been dubbed "the circle of poison." U.S. companies that manufacture these poisons sell them to countries where they are legally sprayed on crops. Then the crops are exported to the United States and are shipped to supermarkets for sale. Ask the store manager where the produce was grown. Armed with this information, you can avoid foods that may be laced with chemicals banned for use in the United States and prevent the most dangerous chemicals from entering your breast milk.

VITAMIN B_{12} AND BREAST MILK

"I'm a vegan. I know I get B_{12} from the fortified breakfast cereals I eat, but am I still shortchanging my son of this important vitamin?"

The only babies at risk belong to breast-feeding moms who eat no animal products whatsoever and who do not eat foods fortified with B_{12} and do not take a B_{12} supplement. However, if you eat eggs or dairy products (which vegans by definition do not include in their diets) or foods fortified with vitamin B_{12}, or pop a multivitamin pill, you have no real worry.

This fat-soluble vitamin is stored in your body, so you don't have to eat it daily for *your* health. But your baby gets the vitamin only from breast milk or an infant formula, not from your body's stores. For his sake, and to be on the safe side, eat your fortified cereal or another B_{12}-containing food every day.

WHEN YOU CAN'T BREAST-FEED

"We're adopting an infant and I don't plan to breast-feed. I worry that my baby girl and I will miss out on the closeness of breast-feeding."

Even when you use bottles, you can provide good nutrition as you snuggle with your baby and provide the blessing of touch, which has lifelong psychological benefits for your baby. It was once believed that bonding had to be immediate or the mother and child would never be truly bonded, but that notion has been disproved. You can develop loving ties with your baby whether she spent her first weeks in an incubator in a hospital's neonatal unit or you first laid eyes on her several months after her birth.

Here are tips:

❖ Start now. When you bring your baby home, spend time getting to know her. Listen to her cries and learn as best you can the difference between "I'm hungry," "I'm wet" and "I want to be held." Most babies crave lots of holding and touching. Some babies who were not held regularly during the first months of life might be hypersensitive to touch at first; talk to your pediatrician for guidance if this is true for your baby.

❖ Get skin-to-skin. Whenever possible, simulate the closeness of breast-feeding by opening your robe or unbuttoning your shirt when you bottle-feed your baby. This isn't possible in public, of course, but make it a priority in private.

❖ Switch arms. A baby gets additional stimulation when she sees the world from your right arm as well as your left. A nursing mom switches arms automatically to empty both breasts. You'll have to make a conscious effort.

❖ Take time. Moms who bottle-feed are more likely than breast-feeding moms to try to get three or more things done at once while their babies eat. When the laundry piles up and you need to get dinner on the table, it's tempting to prop a bottle for your baby and finish chores. But, please, never prop a bottle. Your daughter misses out on the emotional gratification of touch, and she'll be more susceptible to ear infections because of lying on her back while eating.

❖ Instead, hold your baby and caress her. Sing to her (even if you sing off-key) or tell her about your day. When you show her that you love her through touch and attention, she'll learn just how precious she is.

BREAST-FEEDING AN OLDER BABY

"My son is fifteen months old and I plan to breast-feed him until he is at least two years old. I get no support from my family and friends. (Thank goodness my husband is my biggest fan.) Is my intention to breast-feed for longer than average backed by science?"

Breast milk is a good source of nutrition whether your son is one month old or one year old. Studies have shown that breast-feeding has immunological benefits beyond age one, providing him with additional protection against illness. That means he'll get a double benefit: breast milk *and* a vegetarian diet. Breast-feeding also satisfies older babies' suckling needs.

According to La Leche League, in the United States, though a little more than half of mothers nurse their newborns, only 19 percent of six-month-old babies remain at the breast and a mere 5 percent of one-year-olds are breast-fed. Several decades ago, when La Leche League was founded, the common age of weaning was between two and four years old.

The reasons why moms stop or don't try breast-feeding range from sexual connotations associated with the breast to hospital practices encouraging formula feeding (and not supporting breast-feeding) to returning to a workplace where expressing milk is difficult. Just imagine that the only private place to express milk is a bathroom stall.

When few American women breast-feed beyond six months—let alone one year—it's understandable though sad that family members and friends discourage you. Even some psychologists have theorized that breast-feeding an older baby or young child can interfere with psychological development; others have contended, however, that the security that accompanies the closeness of breast-feeding helps children to be independent later in life.

Most important is what you and your husband think. With science on your side, go ahead and breast-feed through your son's second year while ignoring any questioning looks and comments. As long as you and your son are content—and he is thriving—breast-feed to your heart's delight.

PREFERRING FORMULA

"I plan to use infant formula. Tell me the best type to use."

If you choose not to breast-feed, be reassured that your baby can grow up healthy. You just have to supply infant formula that's as scientifically close to breast milk as possible, which all of the major infant formulas are—and to shower your little one with love. Even La Leche League, with its goal of educating and supporting breast-feeding moms, stands behind women who select formula over breast milk if that's the best choice for them.

The two main types of infant formulas on the market are cow's-milk-based formula and soy-based formula. Both supply fats, proteins, carbohydrates, vitamins, minerals and other nutrients in the

---

No Honey!

Don't feed honey to your honey. It may contain the spores of the bacterium *Clostridium botulinum,* which can cause botulism in babies. It is not dangerous to children over one. And since honey is full of empty calories and void of nutrients, it's best eaten sparingly by people of any age.

---

quantities that your baby needs. The main difference between them is their content of either cow's milk or soy.

Though most formulas are made from cow's milk, some babies have trouble digesting the milk protein or are allergic to milk. If this is true for your baby, she may have a constant runny nose, be gassy or have other intestinal troubles. Try switching to a different formula, preferably a soy-based formula, which is made from soybeans. If her runny nose or intestinal troubles clear up within a day or two, it's likely the cow's-milk-based formula was the culprit. A few babies cannot tolerate soy-based formula. Consult your baby's doctor. He or she may recommend a more specialized formula based on your baby's individual needs.

STARTING SOLIDS

"My five-month-old daughter eats her lunch, then suckles for more. Should I start her on solid foods?"

Most babies are ready for solids at about five or six months old; some wait a little longer. Some health practitioners and well-intentioned grandmas favor starting solids as early as possible, but studies suggest that holding off on the spoon may help prevent food allergies and obesity. So before you venture into the wild world of pureed peas and mashed bananas, look for signs of readiness.

One telltale sign is your baby's loss of the tongue thrust reflex. Sticking out her tongue when encountering a foreign object—including food—is a wonderful survival mechanism of a young baby; she automatically pushes out food that could choke her. To check if this reflex has disappeared, place a small amount of a very soft food, such as rice cereal thinned with breast milk or infant formula, or a well-mashed banana, in your baby's mouth. Even if it comes back at you, try a few more times. If she still doesn't take to it, your baby probably isn't ready for solids. Test again in a week or two.

Another sign is her interest in what you're eating. If she's snatching table food or trying to wrestle a fork from you, she's saying that she'd like to try big-people food.

Don't hold off introducing solids too long unless you or your mate has a family history of allergies. A year-old who hasn't tasted anything more exciting than breast milk and a little rice cereal might turn up her nose at even the yummiest peach or mashed potatoes.

There's no one right food to introduce first. Some parents prefer to premier with rice cereal; others favor mashed bananas or pureed vegetables. The one cardinal rule when beginning solids is to introduce only one food at a time for several meals in a row before attempting a second food. The reason is the need to detect any sensitivity to a particular food. If you discover a sensitivity—you may notice diarrhea, gassiness, vomiting, a rash on the face or around the anus, crankiness or a runny nose—discontinue the suspect food. You can try it again in a week or two. If she again shows signs of a sensitivity, keep it out of her diet for a few months before testing it again.

Cereal, vegetables and fruits—and not necessarily in that order—are the foods most babies gobble up eagerly. Don't expect your little one to empty a four-ounce jar of baby food during your first food experimentation or anytime soon. A half teaspoon is plenty. If she seems to want more, offer extra. But don't be surprised or discouraged if the food ends up decorating your baby's face and bib.

After introducing cereal, vegetables and fruits, try whole-grain products, legumes (which are more difficult to digest), cheese and other dairy products, and citrus as well as other potentially highly allergenic foods such as nuts. As she enters her second year, she'll get the majority of her calories from solid foods; milk—whether breast milk, infant formula, cow's milk or soy milk—will account for about sixteen ounces of her food intake. That's a far cry from the thirty-six to forty-eight ounces she slurped up as a young baby.

Studies have confirmed that when you provide a baby or young child with a variety of healthful foods, she invariably selects a wise diet—maybe not at one specific meal, but certainly over the course of a few days. So you supply the nutritious foods and give her freedom to pick and choose. Your baby will grow well with little fuss at all.

A side note: Your attitude shapes your baby's approach to meal-time. A part of her learning about food is seeing what happens when she squishes applesauce between her fingers or flings it on the floor. So practice patience and respect her wishes to end a meal. She knows when she's had enough. To force food on a child teaches her to distrust her own hunger signals and may lead to a lifetime of food problems.

Guidelines for Feeding Your Baby

Roll the video camera. Baby is about to eat her first bite of big-people food. But what's this? She spit out the mashed bananas and it dribbled down her "Gramma Loves Baby" bib?

So goes the typical premier of solids. In the beginning months of solid feedings, more food comes out of your baby's mouth than goes into her tummy. Your baby is learning how to eat. She won't be a pro overnight. That's why breast milk or infant formula remains a vital part of nutrition through your baby's first year of life.

When you start solids, keep a few things in mind:

❖ Schedule meals when your little one is hungry, but not overly hungry, and is in a pleasant mood.
❖ Have the proper equipment: a wiggle-resistant high chair (use the safety buckle); a baby spoon; a big, easy-to-clean bib; clean, damp dish towels for wiping hands and face.
❖ Maintain a sense of humor.

Here's a general guideline to use for starting solids.

Birth to 4 Months

Your baby's nutritional needs can—and should—be met through breast milk or infant formula, unless your child's doctor makes an-other recommendation.

4 to 6 Months

Many babies do not need or want solid foods until they're six months old. When there is a family history of allergies, it's best to wait until she's at least six months old, because an older baby is less likely to develop an allergy to a new food.

If you choose to start solids at four to six months, be sure to try only one food at a time over a few days and watch for any reaction. Discontinue foods that cause reactions. Don't expect your baby to eat more than 1 teaspoon at a meal.

Common foods for this age and beyond:

Mashed ripe banana
Thinned rice cereal
Applesauce
Mashed avocado

Vegetables, cooked and
  mashed
Sweet potatoes
Winter squash
Carrots
Green peas

6 to 8 Months

If you're just starting solids, begin with the foods listed above. Then add these, one at a time:

Thinned oatmeal
Thinned wheat cereal
Fruits, cooked and mashed
  Apples
  Peaches
  Pears

Vegetables, cooked and
  mashed
Green beans
Beets
Broccoli
Cauliflower

As your child accepts various foods, you may serve them at the same meal. Also try finger foods, such as Cheerios, which even toothless babies can gum and swallow quite easily. Be sure the finger foods, such as ripe fresh fruits and well-cooked vegetables, are cut in bite-size pieces. Avoid grapes, which are a choking hazard.

8 to 10 Months

In addition to the foods listed above, you may add:

Baked and mashed potatoes thinned with breast milk or formula
Cubed tofu

Well-cooked legumes
Crackers (avoid the hard varieties)
Fruit juices except citrus

10 to 12 Months

To fill out baby's culinary repertoire, add:

Citrus juices and fruits (unless there is a family history of allergy)
Thinned nut butters
Pasta, cut into bite-size pieces
Bread
Eggs
Other vegetables and fruits that have not yet been introduced

12 months and Beyond

By this time, your child will be eating the same foods you do. You may add milk (cow's or soy), but watch for allergic reactions. Though she may be slurping up milk and eating just like Mom, she probably isn't ready for "adult" meals like stir-fries and casseroles because few kids like mixed-up foods. Just serve her the same ingredients but in separate groupings.

As you might have imagined, starting solids is an adventure. To make it easy on yourself and your little one, expect messes, no table manners and occasional flying food. Before you know it, she'll be reminding *you* not to talk with a mouth full of food.

MEATY QUESTIONS

"Our son is one year old and hasn't tasted meat. The problem is that my in-laws are having Thanksgiving at their home and I know they'll expect their grandson to eat turkey."

Welcome to the uncertain world of proper vegetarian etiquette. What may work in one circumstance or with a specific group of relatives or friends may not apply to other situations or people. Your best bet is planning ahead and being graceful in all circumstances—even if you have to hold your tongue.

First things first. Discuss with your spouse how you both feel about your son eating meat. Some couples will decide firmly against meat eating, while other couples may decide it's okay once in a while, because they may eat meat occasionally too. And still other vegetarian parents may let a young child have a taste and decide for himself.

Then consider the situation. As with most celebrations, food takes center stage. This is especially true on turkey day. Whether turkey ought to be the emphasis is another story. Isn't the giving of thanks as important as, if not more important than, eating turkey?

You also have grandparents in the mix. They've eaten Thanksgiving turkey for more years than they probably care to count and want to carry on tradition. No doubt cranberry sauce, stuffing and pumpkin pie are also part of the food celebration. If you and your son skip the turkey, they might take offense because you're going against not only family tradition but also their values.

The question is, how do you stick to your vegetarian choice with grace?

Loading up your plates with everything but turkey rarely works. A watchful grandparent doesn't miss a trick. Mumbling something about choosing to skip the turkey probably won't succeed either. You're likely to be asked to offer an explanation on the spot or you'll get shot a look that reads: "You hurt my feelings."

The most appropriate, though not necessarily the easiest, step is for you or your spouse to discuss your decision with the grandparents *before* the fourth Thursday in November. State clearly that your family will joyfully eat everything but the turkey on Thanksgiving. Thank them again for their invitation. Tell them what matters most to you is not the menu, but their fine company. That is what you're thankful for.

If they ask questions, respond calmly. The last thing you want to do is give the impression that you don't appreciate them. If necessary, reassure them that their grandson is very healthy indeed. The point is to shift the focus from the turkey to your love for them. Sooner or later—and hopefully sooner—they'll get the message.

"My daughter tasted hamburger at her cousin's house and says she loves it. My wife and I want her to be vegetarian like us. What should we do?"

Before you panic, remember that one taste of hamburger doesn't mean she'll turn into a raving carnivore. You still have almost complete control over her diet at her young age. But as she gets older, she'll insist on having a say too. Many kids of vegetarians remain vegetarian; some don't.

Right now if one of your rules is no meat at home, then so be it. Outside your home is a different story. If your daughter will be at her cousin's house during mealtime in the future, speak to the parent. The parent may not know that meat is off limits for your daughter and will oblige happily by preparing PB&J for her. If not, then you can choose to make sure she isn't at her cousin's house at mealtime. Or invite the cousin to your house, where you serve the meals.

On many occasions during your daughter's childhood, she'll have meat placed in front of her—at a friend's house, during a birthday party or at day care. That gives you many chances to perfect your etiquette skills.

"My husband eats meat and feeds it to our sixteen-month-old when they stop in at fast-food restaurants. I think he's ruining our son's health. He says I'm over-reacting."

It's time to talk—and not only to clearly state to your spouse how you feel but also to listen to his concerns. You *can* come to an understanding by practicing good communication skills. Of course, that's easier said than done.

You do have science on your side, because meat eating is linked to a greater risk of a host of chronic diseases, including heart disease, some cancers, diabetes and obesity. On the other hand, an occasional cheeseburger won't ruin your son's health. If cheeseburgers become a habit, then you have reason for concern.

The landmark Adventist Health Study revealed that vegetarian men live an average of seven years longer than men who regularly eat meat. It was found that part of the increased longevity of vegetarians may be due to lower-fat diets and exercise. Nonetheless, a healthful lifestyle combined with a vegetarian diet is a win-win combo. In fact, figures from the Life Expectancy Reduction Scale by University of Pittsburgh physicist Bernard Cohen, Ph.D., indicate that regularly eating meat sends a man to his grave sooner—yes, sooner—than smoking a pack of cigarettes a day. Smoking shaves off 2,250 days, Cohen calculates, while eating meat steals 2,555 days. (By the way, the Adventist Health Study found that women who eat meat die 7.5 years earlier on average than their vegetarian counterparts, and Cohen calculates that a woman who smokes a pack of cigarettes daily loses 2.2 years of life.)

Talk with your husband about the health advantages of the vegetarian diet and make adjustments as necessary concerning your son's diet. Then get ready to clearly communicate your needs—to your husband or your son—at the next mix-up.

MILK MATTERS

"My pediatrician recommends whole cow's milk for my one-year-old boy, but he seems to have trouble tolerating it."

Because whole cow's milk gets about half of its calories from fat, as does breast milk, the American Academy of Pediatrics and the American Dietetic Association recommend it when a baby weans from breast or bottle. Whether baby humans ought to drink milk designed for baby cows is another question. A minority of physicians say no, citing such reasons as residues of drugs and hormones in cow's milk to the possibility of allergic reaction.

Cow's milk remains the beverage of choice for children and for pregnant and lactating moms. It is a reliable source of calcium, protein and vitamin D (which is added; cow's milk doesn't naturally contain this vitamin), and many people seem to digest milk with little difficulty. There are exceptions, however. After age two to four, members of several ethnic groups—Hispanics, Asians, people of African heritage, and Native Americans—do not produce lactase, an enzyme needed to break down the sugar lactose found in cow's milk. Lactose intolerance, as it's termed, leads to stomach pain, abdominal bloating, gas and diarrhea after drinking milk.

Proteins in cow's milk can be a source of allergy. In fact, it is among the most common food allergens. The symptoms may include stomach pain, diarrhea, nausea, vomiting, hives, rash, ear infections and nasal congestion. They are triggered by the release of histamine in the body in response to the immune system's production of vast numbers of antibodies to attack the food or food component.

To check if cow's milk is the cause of your child's discomfort, remove all dairy products from his diet for several days. If his symptoms disappear, dairy products are the leading suspects. You may choose to feed him dairy products again and note whether the symptoms return. If they do, then your case against dairy products is all but shut tight. Remove the dairy products from his diet again and, if you'd like, test them one at a time, leaving a few days between each test to find out which ones he can tolerate. Sometimes people can eat cheese but not drink milk. Switching from whole cow's milk to 2 percent milk can also make a noticeable difference.

When you drop dairy products from your child's diet, be sure to replace them with a healthful alternative. Soy milk, made from soybeans, tastes similar to cow's milk. The flavor varies from brand to brand, so check out a few of them and select your favorite. Opt for fortified soy milk, which usually has calcium and vitamins D and B_{12} added to it. Once your child reaches his second birthday, switch to a low-fat soy milk. You can also seek out fortified dairy-free milk made from brown rice. At least one brand has as much calcium and vitamins A and D as cow's milk. You'll find dairy-free alternatives to milk in natural food stores and well-stocked supermarkets.

Never feed babies soy milk as a replacement for breast milk or infant formula. Soy milk is deficient in the nutrients a baby needs for proper growth.

"My seventeen-month-old drinks cow's milk like there's no tomorrow. Can he drink too much?

If your son slurps down more than sixteen ounces or so of milk a day, his diet is a bit out of whack. If he's guzzling the white stuff by the quart, make some significant changes in his meals—now.

Eight ounces of milk offer about three hundred milligrams of calcium, eight grams of protein and anywhere from nine grams of fat in whole milk to five grams of fat in 2 percent milk to less than one

---

Homemade Baby Food

Making baby food is as easy as ABC. For a tot adventuring into the world of solids, you'll need the right foods (see "Guidelines for Feeding Your Baby," page 31); a blender, food processor or food mill; ice cube trays; and zip-locked plastic bags. Here are the steps:

1. Cook vegetables and grains until soft, keeping each food separate. Fruits need not be cooked, but be sure to wash them and remove any skins.
2. Place a food in your blender, food processor or food mill and process until completely smooth. This takes a matter of seconds or a few minutes, depending on the food. Using a food mill is the slowest method. Some parents choose to use the food mill only before mealtime, preparing the baby's food from the offerings served to the rest of the family.
3. Spoon your puree into the ice cube trays, place them in the freezer and let freeze.
4. When the food is frozen (this sometimes takes overnight), pop out the cubes and place them in a zipper-type bag. Label the bag—pureed peas and pureed green beans look almost identical—and store them in the freezer for up to three months.
5. At mealtime, remove a cube of food (which equals about two ounces) and warm it up. Make sure not to overheat it or you might burn your baby's mouth.
6. Bring out the spoon and let the fun begin.

gram of fat in skim milk. A glass also delivers about one microgram of vitamin B_{12} and is fortified with vitamins A and D.

Though milk provides ample amounts of certain nutrients, it is lacking in iron and dripping with saturated fat, the kind that can clog arteries, setting the stage for heart disease.

Milk is far from the perfect food that the dairy industry would have you believe. Dairy cows are routinely fed powerful drugs, mostly antibiotics, to treat the infections that have become commonplace at large-scale dairy farms. These drugs have shown up in milk, surveys confirm. The residues can cause reactions ranging from mild skin rashes to severe anaphylactic shock.

Bovine growth hormone (BGH) is also moving into the nation's milk supply. Designed to increase milk production of a dairy cow by 5 to 20 percent, BGH has come under fire from consumers concerned about BGH-tainted milk. Cows given BGH have shown some abnormalities, including reproductive disorders, cardiovascular problems and even premature death, according to the U.S. Food and Drug Administration. Effects on people who drink milk tainted with BGH remain uncertain.

With incomplete nutrition, drug residues and the BGH controversy, milk ought not elbow out better foods from your child's diet. Think whole grains, vegetables, fruits and legumes—and only a limited amount of milk—to make a balanced diet.

TOO MUCH BULK

"Vegetables, fruits and whole-grain breads (the biggest components of our vegetarian diet) contain a lot of fiber. I'm worried that my fourteen-month-old might be getting too much bulk and not enough calories."

Your concern is valid. The tummies of children eating lots of bulky foods fill up before their caloric needs are met. This problem is more common among children who are vegan than among ovo-lacto vegetarian children. Still, studies of vegan kids on a healthful diet show that they develop and grow normally. Vegan kids under five years old tend to be thinner than children eating a diet combining meat and vegetarian foods, but they grow just as tall. The caloric intake of older vegan children is similar to that of nonvegetarians.

Colic Cure?

Your baby has barely made a sound during her first three weeks of life, then wham! She's crying at the top of her lungs. You've checked her diaper and made sure she's not hungry or sick, and she's still crying for hours at a time. Your heart's aching to comfort her.

Sound familiar? Your baby is probably colicky. Colic differs from ordinary crying in that the crying lasts for several hours (and sometimes around the clock), sometimes turns into screaming, and no matter what you try, the crying continues. Many babies clench their fists and pull up their knees. It's estimated that one in five babies suffers from colic.

The reasons for it are not clear. The typical practitioner's prescription seems heartless to parents: Wait it out. But you *can* put matters into your own hands with dietary changes. Though the idea is not widely accepted by pediatricians, changes in your diet if you breast-feed or a switch in your baby's formula sometimes eases colic.

A mom who drinks cow's milk can load her bloodstream with antibodies produced by protein in cow's milk; these antibodies end up in her breast milk and possibly cause colic. Babies fed cow's-milk-based formula may suffer the same result.

The solution: If you breast-feed, stop consuming cow's milk and

---

A child whose diet includes dairy products and eggs will get plenty of fat and sufficient calories. Just avoid the fat-reduced dairy foods and other fat-free products on the market, because children under two need fat for proper growth and development. At two, however, your child should eat a low-fat diet, just like you. Studies have shown that the oft-mentioned guideline of eating no more than 30 percent of calories from fat should be modified. A diet containing no more than 20 to 25 percent of calories from fat is far more healthful, many researchers agree.

dairy products, relying instead on calcium-rich vegetables or a dietary supplement for your nutritional needs. If you use a cow's-milk-based infant formula, switch to a soy-based infant formula. Then note whether the colic lessens in severity or goes away. It just might.

Breast-feeding moms can make other changes. Omit caffeine-containing foods, including your beloved chocolate and your pick-me-up morning cup of coffee. Avoid peanut butter, broccoli, garlic, fish, eggs, carbonated beverages, berries and highly spiced foods; these are known to make some babies fussy.

Certainly, if you haven't already banned tobacco smoke from your house and car, do so now. Though the reason isn't clear, the likelihood of colic increases and the severity worsens when smoke wafts through the air breathed in by an infant. The more smokers in the house, the greater the chance of colic.

Be reassured that the theory linking colic to the inexperience of new moms doesn't hold up under scrutiny: Colic is no less common in babies born to a mom who already has one or more children. Also be aware that colicky babies are not less healthy than their quieter counterparts. In fact, babies who've had colic are just as likely to be healthy and into-everything toddlers. Meanwhile, hang in there. The colic will pass.

Vegan tots need some higher-calorie foods—tofu and other soy foods, avocados and nut butters are excellent choices—to satisfy their energy needs. But don't go overboard: U.S. kids often show the beginnings of atherosclerosis (hardening of the arteries) even before they receive their high school diplomas.

3

Your Toddler

18 Months to 3 Years Old

"No! No! No!" A toddler repeats this word so often—even when she wants the thing she's refusing—that a parent might be driven nuts. Yet she *must* assert herself repeatedly throughout the day to grow and develop. And that brings us into the realm of the kitchen. Realizing that she's a person with ideas of her own, your toddler may turn down—or even toss across the room—the foods that used to be favorites.

She also might say "No!" to meals because she's less hungry and because she's teething. Don't worry if she doesn't finish every meal. Research shows that toddlers who are presented a variety of nutritious foods invariably get enough calories and nutrients for good health.

Your toddler is becoming a social creature with a need for playmates. Though her vocabulary is skyrocketing, anticipate less-than-desirable social skills. She may bite or shove a friend, to your embarrassment. (Don't be overly concerned; almost all kids do it.) This is also the age she'll notice what other kids are eating. If her friends are chomping on bologna sandwiches, she may wonder why she's missing out. Welcome to your first peer-pressure crisis. It won't be your last.

MORE REASSURANCE

"When my boy was just a baby, I didn't think much about nutrition as long as I was breast-feeding and giving him strained vegetables and fruits. Now he's eighteen months old and has the appetite of a horse. Can a vegetarian diet really satisfy not only his hunger but also his nutrition needs?"

A bsolutely. The vegetarian way of eating fits the guidelines of the Food Guide Pyramid, the latest eating guide designed by the U.S. Department of Agriculture. Using a triangle graphic, the Food Guide Pyramid has grains (breads, cereals, rice and pasta) at its base, with a greater number of servings than any of the other food groups. Vegetables and fruit also enjoy a prominent place near the base of the pyramid.

A healthful vegetarian diet emphasizes grains, vegetables and fruits, but it goes a step further. It greatly deemphasizes animal products, especially meats, while the Food Guide Pyramid still promotes these foods. Almost all animal foods overload the body with fat, particularly unhealthful saturated fat (which has been linked to heart disease), and cholesterol. Overwhelming research suggests the vital need to limit the consumption of animal foods.

Another significant and health-promoting difference between the Food Guide Pyramid and the vegetarian diet is that the latter has legumes (rich in protein, iron, fiber and other nutrients) as a staple.

However, both the Food Guide Pyramid and a healthful vegetarian diet put fats, oils and sweets in their proper place by limiting them—except for children under two, who need fat for proper growth and development. (See "In a Fat Fix," page 47.)

Vegetarian toddlers eat many of the foods nonvegetarian kids eat—macaroni and cheese, pancakes, waffles, apple slices, bananas, green beans and peas, to name a handful of delectables. But vegetarian toddlers are more likely than their meat-eating chums to munch on kidney beans and other legumes (wonderful finger foods!) and cubes of tofu. These calorie-dense foods take the place of meat.

Your hungry child needs some calorie-dense foods—including higher-fat foods such as whole milk or fortified soy milk, cheese, full-fat yogurt or soy yogurt, nut butters, avocados and tofu—to provide

---

A Nursery Rhyme Update

When you have a vegetarian child, you'll need to reinvent a few of Mother Goose's favorites. Here's one.

This little piggy went to market.
This little piggy stayed home.
This little piggy had muffins
[or pizza or tofu or any two-syllable kid's food].
This little piggy had none.
And this little piggy went we, we, we, all the way home.

---

ample calories. If your child eats few calorie-dense foods and lots of high-fiber foods, it's quite possible he will feel full *before* his body gets enough calories.

What's important is serving a variety of foods during meals and at snack time. On his plate or high-chair tray, place foods from the various groupings of the Food Guide Pyramid. That means primarily grains (such as whole-wheat bread, cereal, crackers and oatmeal), vegetables, fruits, dairy products or dairy alternatives (such as fortified soy milk and tofu coagulated with a calcium salt—read labels), legumes, eggs if desired, and nuts and seeds. Include vitamin B_{12}-fortified foods if your son eats no animal foods whatsoever. (Vitamin B_{12} is found reliably in animal foods, such as milk and cheese, only.)

FINICKY EATER

''One day my daughter loves PB&J, the next day she pushes it away. And some days it seems that she lives on air. I'm perplexed.''

While toddlers are playing with Legos and dolls, the big people are toying with new ideas to handle finicky eating habits. Studies reassure parents: Children offered a variety of nutritious nibbles get ample calories, vitamins and minerals.

Recognize that toddlers—vegetarian or not—often reject food as a way to assert themselves. If you suspect that your daughter is testing you, take away the unwanted food for a while and try it again in a week. She just might gobble it up. Don't force a "yucky" food on a child. When you make an issue out of food, the child may firmly stand her ground and never eat it again (or at least until she forgets why she stopped eating it in the first place).

Your best strategy is to substitute foods for the ones she doesn't like. If she refuses green vegetables because they taste bitter, offer less bitter-tasting options such as carrots or sweet potatoes. Or try fruit. She might go for apricots, which are high in beta-carotene (the precursor to vitamin A), raisins, oranges, cantaloupe and other vitamin-rich fruits.

If she goes for a day or two eating little food—or "living on air," as you put it—don't worry. Kids are tuned into their hunger—and they *will* eat when they're hungry. Take care to avoid the trap of providing sugary or fatty snacks when they say they want to eat. Instead, offer nutritious snacks. For example, when your daughter skips her juice at breakfast, give her a piece of her favorite fruit as her morning snack, not a fruit roll-up.

Also stay calm when your daughter goes on a "food jag," eating only one or two favorite foods for several days in a row. The body has ample reserves of fat-soluble vitamins—A, D, E and K—and even though the body stores fewer water-soluble vitamins, such as C, there is still a reserve to last a couple of weeks. By that time, her food jag will probably have ended.

However, trust your gut. If you believe your daughter has a health problem, consult a pediatrician or other health practitioner. Though it's unlikely your daughter is sick, learning that she has a clean bill of health will go a long way to reassure you.

DISLIKING VEGETABLES

"My two-year-old son refuses vegetables, even green beans and corn. I'm beside myself."

It can be maddening when your son refuses vegetables of all sorts. But try not to worry. As long as you're providing healthful foods—

Growing Proof

Need more proof that the vegetarian diet is nutritious and satisfying for kids? Consider a landmark study reported in the well-respected medical journal *Pediatrics*. Researchers from the Centers for Disease Control and Prevention examined 404 children raised at the Farm, a Tennessee community that espouses a vegan diet (which contains no animal products whatsoever) and found no significant differences in growth between the vegetarian kids and nonvegetarian kids. On the whole, the vegetarian children were slightly smaller than the American average from ages one to three, then quickly grew to catch up. By age ten, the vegetarian kids were about two and a half pounds lighter and less than one-third of an inch shorter than average.

The next time someone asks whether the vegetarian diet is healthful for kids, answer with a resounding "yes." Then share a few of your favorite recipes.

especially fruits, which are rich in the same nutrients as vegetables—you're doing his body good.

Feel free to be a wee bit sneaky, though. You might try stirring kernels of corn into corn bread or pureeing potatoes and adding the puree to his favorite noodle soup. The puree will make the soup seem creamy. For kids who like some vegetables and not others, you can incorporate a small amount of the disliked vegetable into a dish containing his favorite. A perfect example is mashed potatoes, which most kids like, and broccoli, which many do not. To incorporate the broccoli into the potatoes, first steam the broccoli, then process it in a food processor or blender (or cut it up into very tiny pieces). Stir the broccoli into the potatoes and, with a good measure of aplomb and humor, tell your son that the family is having *green* mashed potatoes for dinner. It might just work.

Another tactic is to provide your son with crunchy, brightly colored raw vegetables, which children seem to prefer over cooked vegetables. When you plan to serve cooked carrots or broccoli to your family, simply set aside some uncooked "pick-up sticks" or "flowers."

Some parents are tempted to give their little ones vitamin supplements. However, once children graduate to solid foods, they don't need vitamin supplements if they're in good health. So says the American Academy of Pediatrics. But if your son not only continues to refuse vegetables but also stops eating fruits and enriched cereals and breads, your pediatrician may recommend vitamin supplements.

IN A FAT FIX

"I've read that kids need more fat than adults. This contention goes against every fiber in my being. I want to make sure my twin girls aren't getting too much fat, setting them up for heart disease and other illnesses down the line."

If your little ones are under two years old, don't skimp on fat. They need this macronutrient for proper growth and development. Children under two also need concentrated calories, and fat has about twice the calories as carbohydrates or protein, gram for gram. If this advice from the National Heart, Lung and Blood Institute, which is supported by the American Academy of Pediatrics, sounds off base, consider this: Breast milk and infant formula (a close approximation of breast milk) both derive about one-half of their calories from fat. Mother Nature knows that your little ones need fat.

But at two years old, your twins ought to switch to a low-fat diet, taking in no more than 30 percent of total calories from fat. Some nutrition researchers say a lower fat intake is better, encouraging a range of 20 to 25 percent of total calories from fat.

Are treats forbidden? Absolutely not. When your children and the rest of the family eat good foods day in and day out, an occasional brownie, cupcake or bag of potato chips is perfectly fine. The goal is healthful eating, not deprivation.

JUNK-FOOD DILEMMA

"My dad loves to give candy to my toddler. I don't want to interfere with their special relationship, but I wish he'd stop doling out junk."

Junk food—whether candy or chicken nuggets—has no place in the everyday diet of a young child or anyone. It's loaded with calories and devoid of nutrition. That said, grandparents have earned special privileges to "spoil" their grandkids. They played the heavy during your childhood. Now it's your turn.

Yet no health-minded parent wants his or her child to fill up on candy and miss out on real meals. Ask yourself a few questions: Is Grandpa doling out candy regularly, say, every day or every few days, or only when he visits twice a year? Is your daughter eating the candy right before meals and ruining her appetite? Is the candy used as a tool to win your daughter's affection?

If the candy handouts are infrequent, aren't spoiling her appetite for lunch or dinner and are an expression of generosity and not a form of manipulation, then seriously consider allowing it. A little candy won't hurt.

But if your dad's behavior is getting under your skin, talk to him and strike a compromise. Suggest treats that you find more appropriate. For instance, cookies sweetened with fruit juice or whole-grain pretzels may fit your idea of healthful alternatives to candy. When your dad understands your dilemma, he's likely to oblige and start handing out healthful treats. Try to be understanding of his motives too. You might find out that you have different ways of expressing the same message: the love for your daughter.

"We've let our son have cookies and cupcakes on occasion. Now he's asking for sweets all the time. Is sugar truly bad?"

Sugar has some sweet and not-so-sweet granules of evidence for and against it. On the positive side, it makes foods taste sweeter—and sweet is favored by children and grown-ups. Research on the whole shows that sugar does not cause cancer, heart disease, diabetes—or hyperactivity, contrary to a commonly held belief.

Though sugar is not a grave health concern, it is something to be reckoned with. Sugar most definitely can cause tooth decay and might suppress the immune system. In addition, sugar is an empty calorie food. It provides no vitamins, no minerals, no fiber. Just calories. Too much sugar may replace nutritious foods in a toddler's limited dietary intake.

Remember, even supposedly more healthful forms of sugar, such as honey, are no better than table sugar. With the exception of black-strap molasses, which provides a significant amount of iron (3.2 milligrams in one tablespoon), sugar in its various forms provides minuscule amounts of nutrients at best. This is why it's wise to limit your child's intake of added sugars.

Offer alternatives to sugary snacks. The ideal is fruit. Other options are sweetened breads and cookies that contain some nutrition. Examples are banana bread, preferably made with whole-wheat flour, carrot-raisin muffins and oatmeal cookies. Keep snacks like candy bars to a minimum. And be a good role model. If you rarely eat sweets and don't keep them in your home, your child will probably follow your lead.

But take a *psychological* approach to sugar: Parents who ban it completely might find their child's interest in sweet stuff heighten exponentially. The child's thinking goes something like this: "I must be missing out on something fun if my mommy says no." So say yes once in a while.

No!

"Whenever I try a new food, or a new combination of foods, I keep hearing 'No!'"

When mealtime becomes a battlefield, common sense and compromise must prevail. First, remember that "No!" may not mean your little one dislikes the food. It often means that your naysayer is trying to exert some control.

On one hand, the realization of his personhood is a good thing, paving the way toward healthy self-esteem. On the other hand, if a child learns that his mom or dad will bend over backward to placate his every whim, the child might learn the art of manipulation all too well.

The Best Healthful Snacks

Fruits of all sorts, including banana chunks, apple slices, orange
  sections, grapes cut in half (whole grapes are a choking hazard),
  kiwi slices, melon chunks, raisins and other favorites
Fresh vegetables, such as broccoli florets and carrot and celery sticks
Whole-grain crackers
Whole-grain pretzels
Fruit muffins
Rice cakes smeared with jam or nut butter
Cheerios, Kix or another low-sugar cereal that's easy to pick up
  with fingers
Cheese cubes
Fruit-flavored yogurt
Tofu cubes
No-oil tortilla chips
Air-popped popcorn
Low-fat cookies
Sorbet
Rice-based frozen dessert

The best approach, nutrition and child-care experts agree, is to
realize that toddlers—vegetarians and meat eaters—are notorious for
saying no even to foods they like. They also tend to resist new foods
and combinations of foods. (Do you recall the days when you went
into a frenzy at the mere sight of green peas touching your mashed
potatoes?)

With this realization, use common sense when introducing
foods. One tried-and-true method is to place a small spoonful of the
new food on his plate and allow him a "no thank you" bite. He tests
the food but knows he won't be pressured into eating more of the
new food. Sometimes the child discovers he likes his first taste and
asks for more. Don't pressure your son to eat normal portions of new
foods; such tactics usually backfire, with your son clenching his jaw
and possibly throwing a temper tantrum.

When making a combination dish for your family (examples include casseroles, tacos and even sandwiches), keep in mind that many toddlers do not like mixed-up foods. You can still provide a nutritious meal made up of the mixed-up foods; just don't mix them up. For instance, if bean tacos are on the menu, set aside a portion of beans, a broken-up taco shell and piles of tomato, lettuce and cheese on your child's plate. This way you don't have to make an extra meal—and what parent wants to be a short-order cook anyway?

CLEANING THE PLATE

"Now that our son is older, my wife tries to get him to finish everything on his plate. She wants to instill the value of not wasting food. But once he's had enough, he insists on getting out of his high chair. Dinnertime is becoming a boxing match."

A t almost all costs, do what you must to make dinnertime pleasant. Stress is bad for digestion, and your child learns life lessons about food at an early age. With that in mind, your wife ought to be commended for her desire to not waste food. However, it's bad judgment to require a child to clean his plate.

Many parents have prompted children to finish every morsel because children in India or Zimbabwe or Haiti are starving. Though many children in the world do starve—a sad truth, to be sure—it's fallacy that an American kid who cleans his plate prevents starvation. In fact, overeating is a waste. Truly, when you eat more calories than your body requires, you've wasted food.

A better approach is serving smaller portions to your son. Then if he asks for more, give him an extra spoonful or two. This way food waste is kept to a minimum. Also remember that toddlers have small tummies that fill up quickly. Don't expect him to eat big meals. Rather, plan on several nutritious snacks during the day.

Combining the desire to not waste food with maintaining a realistic view of kids' typical (which might seem crazy) eating habits is a win-win proposition.

VEGE-WHAT?

"When is a good time to tell my boy that he's a vegetarian?"

In a home where one or both parents are vegetarian, the v-word is bound to come up now and then. The word will become part of his vocabulary, though he's likely to mispronounce it at first. He even may exclaim to family and friends that he's a *veterinarian*.

Being vegetarian is a fact of his life that he'll accept, no questions asked. At first. As your child heads into his preschool years, he'll question why the kid down the block eats turkey sandwiches and he doesn't. Or he may wonder why you don't take him to McDonald's for a Happy Meal when many of his friends make frequent fast-food visits.

When your son starts asking questions—or when it seems that he's ready to hear a brief description of the word *vegetarian*—be ready to offer an explanation. Keep your language simple. As you know, your child will more likely listen and understand your answers when they are age-appropriate.

Try a definition along these lines: "Vegetarians are people who don't eat meat, chicken or fish [or eggs and dairy foods, if you're vegan] but who eat every other yummy food. Some animals, including giraffes, cows and brontosaurus, are (or were) vegetarian, too." Stress the value of differences and that it's okay for friends to eat differently. What a person eats doesn't make him or her good or bad, just unique.

You might want to tell your child why you're vegetarian, again keeping the language simple. You could say that you're a vegetarian because it helps keep you strong and healthy. Or you might say that you love animals and don't want to eat them. Most important, be honest and gentle. Then your little one will get the message that you love him as he is—vegetarian or not.

TROUBLE WITH RELATIVES

"When we visit my mom around noon, she insists on serving us lunch. But she has only white bread (never whole wheat), cold cuts and chips on hand. I don't want my daughter eating that stuff. What do I say to my mother?"

That depends. Would you risk your relationship with your mother if you have a heart-to-heart talk with her about your daughter's diet? Does the knowledge that your little one is eating meat and junk food sicken you? Before you approach your mother, weigh the costs of the possible outcomes.

Food habits die hard. If your mother thinks white bread, meat and junk food are acceptable fare, she probably won't change her mind. She also might think your dietary choices for your daughter mean that you don't value or respect her. However, during an honest talk with your mother, you can dispel any wrong notions she might have about your feelings toward her by your telling her that you do, in fact, love and esteem her. You can also appeal to her love for her granddaughter as a sound reason to serve her more nutritious foods.

Offer to bring your own lunches and snacks to your mom's house. She might take you up on your offer or decide to buy nutritious nibbles on her own. When you let your mother know that you want to help her while you do what's best for your daughter, she'll see that your heart is pure.

"My in-laws can't understand why we're raising our children as vegans. They think the kids will be irreversibly harmed."

Your in-laws' concern is not surprising. Even though most research backs up a vegan diet that offers variety, some studies have zeroed in on a few isolated cases in which a child or a few children were malnourished and blamed the vegetarian diet.

Tell your in-laws that you are careful to feed foods that provide all of the nutrients their grandchildren require. The proof is the children. If you are indeed offering a varied diet and are aware that vegan kids need fortified foods that provide vitamin B_{12}, which occurs reliably in animal foods only, their regular checkups will show that they are growing and are in good health.

Some people dismiss a vegan diet no matter what you say or how many medical reports you show them. In such cases, your best bet is to remain confident that you're making healthful decisions for your children and to thank your in-laws for their concern.

The Dairy Dilemma

"Drink your milk, honey." Millions of moms and dads have uttered these words. But is their instruction good advice?

Though cow's milk is a rich source of calcium, the creamy stuff has come under fire. When a 1989 *Wall Street Journal* investigation turned up drug residues in about 40 percent of milk samples from ten major cities, the findings made headlines.

But the situation hasn't changed since then. Contaminants like antibiotics still remain in the milk supply. In some sensitive people, these drugs can cause reactions as mild as hives or as serious as anaphylactic shock. Now newer drugs like bovine growth hormone (BGH) are being fed to dairy cows to increase their milk production.

Some renegade health practitioners discourage people from drinking milk. They point not only to health reasons but also to common sense: Cow's milk is meant for calves, not boys and girls.

SURVIVING THE HOLIDAYS

"When I used to go to my parents' home for Christmas or the Fourth of July, I picked around the meat and usually nobody said anything. Now the relatives ask me why my daughter's plate is missing the meat. I wish I could just disappear into the wallpaper."

When your child graduates to big-people food, relatives will notice what she eats. That's a given. So are the questions that'll follow: Aren't you going to give her meat? Where is she going to get her protein? Aren't vegetarian diets bad for children? And on and on.

The trick is to handle as many of these questions as possible in advance of the holiday party. Tell the host something like, "We're delighted to accept your dinner invitation. Our daughter is looking forward to the party. She doesn't eat meat, so please don't take offense when we fill up her plate with your other lovely dishes."

If the host asks why she's a vegetarian, be honest. Say that a vegetarian diet is healthful for children as well as adults and that the

American Dietetic Association and the American Academy of Pediatrics also support meatless diets for kids.

By breaking the news to your host, other relatives may learn of your daughter's diet and won't ask so many questions. And if they do grill you, don't be afraid to speak boldly yet with a good measure of humor and love. Most people who become vegetarian have learned about it from a friend or family member. Think of yourself as a bearer of good tidings.

BIRTHDAY PARTIES

"My vegetarian son has been invited to his three-year-old friend's birthday party. Hot dogs are on the menu."

Many vegetarian parents who find their children in this situation allow them to eat whatever is on the menu—hot dogs, chocolate cake and punch included. They view this detour from the family's usual diet as acceptable because it's a once-in-a-while occurrence.

At three years old and older, most children are acutely aware if they are singled out. They *want* to eat what everyone else is eating. If it's any consolation, young children are usually too excited at a birthday party to eat much food anyway.

If you know the party givers fairly well, you could ask them to give your son a PB&J sandwich instead of a hot dog. However, a better idea might be to feed your son some lunch before he goes to the party and tell him to eat the cake but skip the hot dog, because he's already eaten.

Don't expect this birthday party "problem" to go away anytime soon. You and your son will have many more opportunities, as he gets older and receives more invitations to birthday parties, to dream up new, creative solutions to this sticky situation.

"We're having some kids over for our daughter's birthday party. She'll be three. What's a workable menu that everyone will like?"

When your child is the birthday girl, you get to plan the menu. Omitting meat causes no problem. Toddlers gobble up cheese pizza, PB&J sandwiches (especially when cut into fun shapes with cookie cutters) and noodles with delight. Realistically, toddlers and preschoolers are so excited by the party festivities that their platefuls of food go almost uneaten.

In planning the birthday menu, keep in mind the theme of the party: teddy bears, tea party, dinosaurs, a Disney character or whatever appeals to your daughter. Plan the menu accordingly. For example, you could make open-faced peanut butter sandwiches cut into bear shapes with a cookie cutter (place raisins on the face for eyes and a nose) and serve some apple slices or melon balls on the side. Offer juice as the beverage.

You could carry on the teddy bear theme by making a cake in the shape of a bear. Or place small teddy bears cut from brown paper bags on the cake with the use of toothpicks. Be sure to place them away from where the candles will go, for obvious reasons. In choosing a cake, you could go decadent or healthful, depending on your preference. In the recipe section in the second half of this book, you'll find healthful options.

Most important, keep the food simple, fun to eat and easy to clean up. Expect a few spills. (Place a disposable plastic tablecloth *under* the table and chairs, especially if you have carpeting, to simplify cleanup.) You'll be too busy running games and helping your child open gifts to spend lots of time in the kitchen.

CHILD CARE

"Our twenty-two-month-old is in a day-care home. To our satisfaction, the caregiver has agreed to feed only healthful vegetarian lunches and snacks to our daughter. The problem is that the other kids eat meat lunches and sugary desserts. Will our child feel left out?"

A child younger than two eats what's in front of her without much thought to what the other kids are gobbling up—unless the caregiver makes a big deal out of your daughter's meal and snacks. If the caregiver points out the difference, then the other kids will notice too, and she may feel left out. It's important to talk with the caregiver and inquire about how she handles mealtime.

Snacks are more likely to be an issue when your daughter notices

How to Get Good Food at Day Care

With most parents working outside the home and their young children spending significant time in day care (including lunch and two snacks daily), it's wise to enroll your kids at a day-care center that respects—and even reflects—your food preferences.

Only a very small percentage of day-care centers will offer a vegetarian meal or option every day. It's far more likely that a center will provide cheese slices or a peanut butter and jelly sandwich in place of the main entrée; cheese and PB&J every weekday can get boring fast. Some centers won't even go this far.

The number-one rule: Ask questions about the center's food policies *before* you plunk down the first week's tuition.

You might be allowed to pack a lunch for your kids. This means more work for you, of course, but you'll have the peace of mind that your children are eating well. Expect some surprises, though. Toddlers are notorious for swiping food from other children's plates. Call it keen curiosity.

Take an active role in your children's day-care center. You might be able to influence the menu. For example, especially if you have other parents on your side, you might convince the day-care center to include more vegetarian entrées in a given week's menu. Or you might talk the day-care director into serving meatballs on the side when spaghetti with tomato sauce is on the menu. You also might make inroads in improving the overall healthfulness of the day's menu by suggesting more vegetables and fruits and fewer fatty foods.

Another tack is signing up your children at a Montessori or Waldorf school, both of which are generally accepting of vegetarian kids and their parents. Check your yellow pages.

she's not receiving the same brightly packaged, sugary snacks as the other kids. Encourage the caregiver to provide tasty nibbles like pretzels, air-popped popcorn, lightly sweetened rice cakes, fruit and fairly benign cookies such as vanilla wafers to *all* of the children. Consider bringing the caregiver a package of snacks to share with everyone.

Then your child will feel she's one of the gang—and you'll help to improve the quality of the snacks for her friends too.

As your daughter heads toward her three-year-old birthday, you'll notice that she is probably more greatly keyed into what her friends are eating at lunch. Now's the time she might feel left out if she's not permitted to eat bologna sandwiches like everyone else. Depending on your feelings, you may decide to allow her to eat the meals served by the caregiver while encouraging the caregiver to of-fer vegetarian lunches (spaghetti with tomato sauce and pancakes, to name two examples) some of the time.

Gently ask your child how she feels. If she wants to try meat at day care, consider allowing it. Or you can stand firm, and tell your child that she won't have meat because that's a family rule. If you take the latter approach, be consistent. Otherwise, your child may think you'll change your mind if she complains loud enough. With either approach, you have assurance that when she's home, you feed her the very best foods.

"What should we tell a new baby-sitter about our three-year-old's diet?"

When a new baby-sitter is serving meals or snacks to your tod-dler, let him or her know clearly which foods are permissible and which are not. An almost foolproof method is to prepare the meals and snacks in advance, with accompanying heating directions, if appropriate.

Also tell the baby-sitter about any mealtime rituals—such as which chair your child uses, favorite plates and bowls, a prayer you might say before eating—that you'd like to be retained for the time you're away. Another approach is suggesting to the baby-sitter to do something out of the ordinary, such as having an indoor picnic or serving a big bowl of popcorn while watching a video. That way your child's guaranteed a good time with her new baby-sitter.

4

Your Preschooler
3 to 5 Years Old

Full of curiosity, your preschooler is becoming less me-centered as he takes a greater interest in the world around him. He turns over rocks in search of bugs, delights in watching shoots turn into flowers and makes mud pies. His active imagination turns him into a superhero by day and a frightened child at night when shadowy monsters are on the loose.

Kids have a natural affinity toward animals, so feel free to talk about their inherent value. Also discuss where meat comes from and why your child is a vegetarian. Your supportive words will come in handy as he faces situations where meat is served: birthday parties, holiday get-togethers, lunches at friends' houses and so on. He is sensitive to his peers' comments and may want to try meat. How you handle this challenge is a purely personal decision. Some parents make meat off limits; others permit their child to taste it.

Whatever your decision, be sure to emphasize the fact that good foods help him grow. Teach him which foods are best. And because your preschooler eagerly takes in new information and wants to please you—at least most of the time—you have an ideal forum for talking about nutrition. Take advantage of the opportunity.

NUTRITION 001

"My little girl asks zillions of questions and wants answers to everything. Now seems like a ripe time to teach her the facts about good nutrition."

A preschooler hungry for knowledge won't be denied. She'll ask questions from sunup until sundown, expecting answers. If she's asking questions about food, great. Your work is half done. If she isn't, you can plant the seed by having her join in the cooking or gardening and talking to her about food.

In either case, seize this opportunity to teach her about good nutrition. A good place to start is her body and how it works. Get your hands on a kid-friendly book that shows the parts of the body, from the skeleton and the muscles to the lungs and the digestive tract. Tell her that good food helps her body grow and gives her energy.

You also might name superheroes who become strong when they eat well. Popeye, the champ of spinach, is the first to come to mind. (Whether the sailor man ought to gulp down his leafy greens is another matter altogether.) But be prepared when she says pepperoni pizzas must be healthful because the Teenage Mutant Ninja Turtles eat them by the case load. Thankfully, the Turtles are no longer "in," but she might see TV reruns or old videos.

You'll need to help her differentiate between good food and junk food. Use television commercials and magazine advertisements as teaching tools. Tell her that some foods look fun but are loaded with sugar, fat and other yucky stuff. Inform her that product manufacturers are trying to snooker her into desiring what they're selling. They want to make money; few are interested in her well-being.

When she asks specific questions about food, such as "Why is cantaloupe orange?" give answers appropriate to her age. To this question, for instance, you might say something like, "Cantaloupe is orange because it has lots of beta-carotene. That's a vitamin that helps keep you healthy and strong. Carrots also have beta-carotene." You get the idea.

Most of all, remember that your actions speak louder than words. If you want your daughter to eat well, then make good food choices for yourself and the entire family. Follow wise eating habits too.

These include sitting while you eat, chewing well and eating when hungry. Children learn their lifelong eating habits early on. Your daughter is off to a great start. Congratulations.

GROWING UP

"Compared to other kids her age, my four-year-old daughter looks skinny and small. She's been a vegetarian since birth. Have I done something wrong?"

P robably not. A child's size is determined by heredity and less so by nutrition. If you've fed your little girl adequate calories and a variety of foods, she is probably the epitome of health, petite or not.

A good guideline to monitor her growth is the one health practitioners use: If she continues to get taller and gain weight season after season, even though she's smaller than other four-year-olds in your neighborhood, she's doing fine. However, if her growth has slowed dramatically or if you suspect a health problem, consult your pediatrician or other practitioner to assess her health—and ease your fears.

You might hear from well-meaning friends and relatives that your daughter's vegetarian diet is the cause of her petite stature. But listen to the studies:

A landmark study of children reared at the Farm, a Tennessee community espousing a vegan diet (free of all animal products, even cow's milk), showed no significant differences in height and weight from the average U.S. youth population. In a separate study by researchers at Loma Linda University in California, vegetarian kids measured up again. In the two-year study of 2,272 children aged six to eighteen, researchers compared the heights and weights of Seventh-Day Adventist schoolchildren to their public school counterparts. (About one-half of Seventh-Day Adventists, who adhere to a biblical teaching that the body is the temple of the Holy Spirit, are vegetarian, but even those who eat meat tend to eat less of it than the average American.) The study's findings: Girls of similar age showed no significant difference in height, but Adventist boys were, on average, 1.6 centimeters (about five-eighths of an inch) *taller* than their peers. Both Adventist boys and girls were leaner than the non-

Adventists. These findings led the Loma Linda University researchers to conclude that a healthful lifestyle, including a vegetarian diet, supports optimal physical growth.

So as long as your daughter is growing, don't worry. She'll reach the height programmed by her genes in the decade to come.

WEIGHTY CONCERNS

"My preschooler is chubby. I'd hate to put him on a diet, but I don't want him to end up fat."

Diets for little kids make little sense—especially when you have other options. Before looking at some slim-down strategies, consider these points:

First, even though your son seems chubby to you, he might be of optimal weight for his height. Check with your pediatrician or other health practitioner. Second, preschoolers have growth spurts. His chubbiness might disappear on its own without any changes in his diet when he shoots up a few inches in the months to come. Third, body size is inherited. If you or your spouse tends to be big-boned and stocky, your son might end up looking like a linebacker too.

But because early signs of heart disease can show up in young children—an elevated blood cholesterol level, for instance—it's wise to feed kids good-for-the-heart foods from day one. This is especially true in families in which heart disease has claimed victims. By feeding your son good foods, you'll set the stage for healthful eating. Be careful not to overload your son's meals with cheese and eggs, a common mistake among many new and some veteran vegetarians. The bulk of the diet ought to be plant foods.

If you decide to slim down your son's diet, the best approach isn't an eating plan that restricts certain foods and requires him to eat other foods he might detest. A better way is improving the entire family's food choices. This might mean ridding your cupboards of cookies and chips. Or perhaps you'll need to trade in your high-fat dessert recipes for low-fat alternatives (baked apples in place of apple pie, for instance). The point is to lower the fat content of the family's meals in general. Your son won't feel singled out.

Another strategy is to keep the serving dishes in the kitchen and out of the dining area at mealtime. Studies have shown that diners are more likely to take second helpings when a tray of food is sitting right in front of them. Instead, place a reasonable portion on each diner's plate. If anyone is still hungry, he or she can ask for another helping.

Be careful not to fall into the trap of serving snacks to kids who haven't eaten a good meal. Kids are notorious for eating a little at lunch or dinner and then requesting crackers or cookies only minutes after mealtime. A way to handle this situation is to tell a child who's barely touched his meal that if he gets hungry, he can finish his meal and that he won't receive a snack. When you follow through on your promise, he'll start to eat the good foods you serve at mealtime.

By combining low-fat meals and using some strategies that discourage overeating—and encouraging exercise in the form of children's play (bike riding, hide-and-seek, building snow friends, to name a few)—you will probably watch your child's chubbiness melt away without having to resort to a restrictive diet, which almost always fails.

LOADING UP ON CARBS

"We eat tons of pasta, grains and bread at our home. I've heard conflicting reports on the value of a diet high in carbohydrates."

Carbohydrates are nutritional royalty. Consider this: A classic experiment carried out at the end of World War II clearly demonstrated that children will develop normally on a diet consisting of plenty of bread and vegetables with minimal amounts of milk and meat. Bread was the mainstay of the children's diet and they thrived.

More proof in the bread pudding: The Food Guide Pyramid designed by the U.S. Department of Agriculture has grains (bread, cereal, rice and pasta) at the base of the pyramid, recommending six to eleven servings a day. These foods provide complex carbohydrates (sometimes called starches), which are the body's most important source of energy. Without them, your child would be running on empty. Complex carbohydrates are also a good source of dietary fiber.

The main controversy over carbohydrates is the rehashed concern that they are fattening. No way, say dietitians. Carbohydrates have four calories per gram compared to the nine calories per gram in fat. The problem is adding fat to high-carbohydrate foods. Examples are butter slathered on bread, sour cream mounded on baked potatoes and cheese sauce poured over pasta.

The upshot: Stick with the Food Guide Pyramid's recommended number of servings, while keeping in mind that a child's portion is about one-half that of an adult portion, and eat carbohydrates to your heart's content.

MORE ON PROTEIN

"How do children's needs for protein change as they grow?"

As children get taller and put on weight, they need to consume more protein. Your little ones will need an extra boost of protein when they hit adolescence and experience the body changes that come with puberty. But relax: Getting adequate protein is no problem, for several reasons.

The most obvious reason is that as kids grow, their appetites increase, so they consume more food and thereby get more protein. A second reason is that the body manufactures some of its own protein. More specifically, only nine amino acids (or building blocks of protein) are not made by the body and must be consumed in the diet.

Contrary to common belief, almost all foods contain enough of each amino acid, so that if your child ate nothing but rice, which is low in the amino acid lysine, he still wouldn't court a protein deficiency, as long as he was getting enough calories. Of course, you wouldn't feed your child only one food. A single food cannot meet all of the nutrient needs of the body. (For more on the protein myth, see "Protein—How Much for Good Health?" page 16.)

A third reason is that getting adequate protein takes little effort. In fact, surveys show that most Americans, including vegetarian children, consume *more* protein than they need.

Let's take a look at the recommended dietary allowance (RDA) for protein, which nutrition experts generally agree is right on target.

The RDA for protein for children aged one to three is sixteen grams daily; for children aged four to six, twenty-four grams daily; and for children aged seven to ten, twenty-eight grams daily. For girls aged eleven to fourteen, the RDA for protein is forty-six grams daily, then it drops to forty-four grams and increases again to forty-six grams from ages nineteen to twenty-four. From age twenty-five onward, the protein need for women is fifty grams daily.

For boys aged eleven to fourteen, the RDA for protein is forty-five grams daily, then it increases to fifty-nine grams daily from age fifteen to eighteen, drops to fifty-eight grams from nineteen to twenty-four, and remains at sixty-three grams daily for the rest of their lives.

The recommended dietary allowances are exactly that: recommendations. They are not minimum requirements. So stop worrying: Your growing kids get plenty of protein.

TOO LITTLE IRON?

"I'm concerned about my daughter's iron intake and whether she might become anemic, even though she eats a healthful vegetarian diet. If she isn't eating meat, how does she get enough iron?"

Iron from plant foods, such as legumes, dried fruits and dark leafy greens, are not as readily absorbed as the iron in meat. However, vegetarian kids tend to take in generous amounts of vitamin C, which enhances iron absorption. In effect, this means their iron status is as good as, if not better than, the iron status of meat-eating kids, research shows.

Studies evaluating iron levels in vegetarians found no evidence of increased iron deficiency—unless the diet was very restricted. As you know, a healthful vegetarian diet comprises a variety of foods, including iron-rich taste treats. (See "Iron-Rich Foods," page 13.) The recommended dietary allowance for iron is ten grams daily for children aged six months to ten years.

Chances are your vegetarian daughter will never have low iron stores, because she's eating well. Iron-deficiency anemia is the most common type of anemia. When a person is deficient in iron, her red blood cells remain small and pale and do not mature properly.

Curiously, eating too much iron may increase cancer risk. A study of 8,500 American men and women found that the risk of developing cancer began to rise when the level of iron in the study participants' blood was just 10 percent above average. The reason for the iron-cancer link is unclear.

MICRONUTRIENTS

"Phosphorus, magnesium, zinc—these nutrients confuse me. Should I be concerned how much of each one my three-and-a-half-year-old is getting through his diet?"

C arbohydrates, protein, fat and fiber are called macronutrients because the body needs them in large quantities. (Saying you need fat in a large quantity sounds heretical, but relatively speaking, your body needs far more fat than vitamins and minerals.) Micronutrients, such as the ones named in the question plus selenium, copper and many others, are required in minuscule amounts. Yet they are essential to good health.

There is a lot about micronutrients that researchers do not know—so you are not alone in your confusion. Don't get hung up on individual micronutrients because you might do damage to your little one. You see, an excessive intake of any single micronutrient can cause a nutritional imbalance. If a person ate lots of zinc, he might deplete his copper stores because these two micronutrients are interrelated. The same is true for other micronutrients.

Your best bet is to focus on the big picture. When your child is eating a healthful diet, he will undoubtedly get the proper amounts of the various micronutrients.

CHEWABLE VITAMINS

"I'm tempted to buy chewable vitamins for my four-year-old. On some days she eats her fruits and vegetables. On other days she wants only bread and cheese."

When a child goes on a food jag, eating one or two foods meal after meal for several days straight, or if a parent of a well-rounded eater just wants extra insurance, chewable vitamins seem a reasonable solution.

However, the American Academy of Pediatrics says your child doesn't need the extra nutrients, assuming she's eating a reasonable diet. But if your child eats no dairy products or eggs, she ought to receive a reliable source of vitamin B_{12}. You can turn to fortified foods, such as some breakfast cereals and soy milk, or you could give her a B_{12} supplement.

Just be careful not to monkey around with single nutrients without approval from your pediatrician or other health practitioner. Overdoing a vitamin or mineral can cause nutritional imbalances.

If you choose to give your child a multivitamin or other supplement, you'll find a wide selection in drugstores and natural food stores. Some brands in natural food stores avoid artificial colors, artificial flavors, sweeteners and preservatives. As with any drug, keep vitamins out of the reach of children.

MORE ON JUNK FOOD

"We cleaned up our diet only after my preschoolers had more than their share of junk food. They miss their old favorites and complain. Can we really turn back now without too many fights?"

Don't pull out your boxing gloves yet. You can rid your preschoolers' diets of junk food without resorting to fighting. You just need a few tricks up your sleeve. Here are some ideas.

❖ Don't completely ban junk food. A forbidden food takes on a special aura of intense desire. If your children are never allowed favorite treats now and then, they might gobble up junk food at Grandma's condo or at friends' houses and eat it in greater quantity than had you permitted it in your home.

❖ Talk to your children about the pros and cons of junk food (it may taste good, but other foods are better for your body). Tell them that because you want the best for them, you plan to limit the

Supervitamins

Vitamins that pack a powerful nutritional punch are C, E and beta-carotene, all of which are antioxidants. The antioxidants are becoming household words as scientists learn more about these immune boosters and publish books about them.

To make a long story short, antioxidants are substances that neutralize free radicals, which are chemical agents that can lead to disease. Free radicals are chemically very reactive because they are molecules with an unpaired electron. They swipe electrons from stable molecules, turning them into new free radicals that in turn prey on other molecules. The resulting cellular damage can translate into disease. Scientists have linked some sixty diseases to free radicals, including cancer and heart disease.

Antioxidants render free radicals harmless by either taking away or donating electrons, thus eliminating the unpaired electron. Though the body produces its own antioxidants, vitamins C, E and beta-carotene (the precursor to vitamin A) lend a helping hand in the battle against free radicals.

A healthful vegetarian diet overflows with these vitamins. Here are some rich sources:

amount of junk food they eat. Then stand firm. Children start whining and whimpering when they think you'll buckle under their pressure.

❖ Take a gradual approach—unless you sense your kids are ready to go cold turkey. Most children like to get used to a new family rule. They need time to adjust. Get rid of the junkiest foods first. Candy bars, ice cream, soft drinks and potato chips ought to go. Then make further eliminations: french fries, fruit roll-ups, fatty crackers and cookies and other foods you consider too junky to keep in the house.

❖ At the same time you're eliminating junk foods, add other foods to your snack cabinet. You might buy cookies sweetened with fruit

Vitamin C:
Broccoli (½ cup chopped, raw): 41 milligrams (mg.)
Brussels sprouts (4 sprouts, boiled): 48 mg.
Grapefruit (½ medium): 47 mg.
Kiwi (1 medium): 75 mg.
Orange (1 medium): 80 mg.
Potato (1 medium, baked, with skin): 26 mg.
Strawberries (1 cup): 85 mg.

Vitamin E:
Almonds (24 nuts): 6.7 mg.
Hazelnuts (1 ounce): 6.7 mg.
Peanut butter (1 tablespoon): 3 mg.
Safflower oil (1 tablespoon): 4.6 mg.
Wheat germ (¼ cup): 6 mg.
Whole wheat (⅓ cup): 3 mg.

Beta-carotene:
Cantaloupe (1 cup pieces): 516 retinol equivalents (RE)
Carrot (1 medium, raw): 2,025 RE
Kale (½ cup chopped, boiled): 481 RE
Mango (1 medium): 806 RE
Papaya (1 medium): 612 RE
Pumpkin (½ cup mashed, boiled): 2,691 RE
Sweet potato (1 medium, baked): 2,488 RE

juice, baked tortilla chips, whole-wheat pretzels, frozen fruit juice bars, flavored rice crackers and other healthful alternatives to junk food. Also keep easy-to-grab vegetables and fruits in your refrigerator. Celery and carrot sticks, broccoli florets (or baby trees), grapes, watermelon chunks and orange slices are quite enticing when they're prewashed and kept on a low shelf in the refrigerator. You can also make healthful snacks, such as low-fat muffins and cookies.

❖ When your kids are invited to a birthday party for cake and ice cream or if they have a hankering for chips and dip, consider suspending the family rule about junk food. Remember, as long as your children's usual diet is healthful, a little junk won't hurt them.

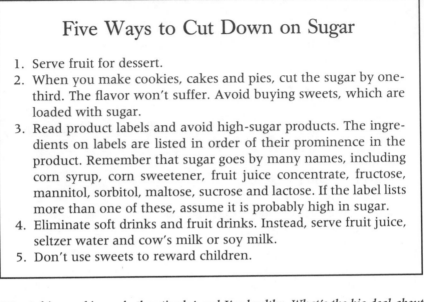

Five Ways to Cut Down on Sugar

1. Serve fruit for dessert.
2. When you make cookies, cakes and pies, cut the sugar by one-third. The flavor won't suffer. Avoid buying sweets, which are loaded with sugar.
3. Read product labels and avoid high-sugar products. The ingredients on labels are listed in order of their prominence in the product. Remember that sugar goes by many names, including corn syrup, corn sweetener, fruit juice concentrate, fructose, mannitol, sorbitol, maltose, sucrose and lactose. If the label lists more than one of these, assume it is probably high in sugar.
4. Eliminate soft drinks and fruit drinks. Instead, serve fruit juice, seltzer water and cow's milk or soy milk.
5. Don't use sweets to reward children.

"I eat chips, cookies and other 'junk,' and I'm healthy. What's the big deal about snacking?"

Snacking is good for preschoolers. They need an extra boost of nutrition between mealtimes. The question is, what type of snacks rank high in nutrition? Not chips, cookies and other "junk." These score points for sugar and fat. Over time, poor eating translates into disease. Five of the ten deadliest diseases in America are diet-related. So says a U.S. Surgeon General report. Though you might not see the ravaging effects of a bad diet yet, you're playing with fire.

Rethink your approach to snacking and teach your child to choose good foods. You won't regret it.

WHEN SPOUSES DISAGREE

"I recently cut meat out of my diet. I want to raise my child as a vegetarian, but my husband (who eats meat) says I shouldn't bother. Where can I find support?"

So-called mixed marriages can be trying. When one spouse is a vegetarian and the other one isn't, finely tuned communication

How Sweet Is Sugar?

Let's bury a myth: White table sugar (the chemical name is sucrose) is no worse for you than are brown sugar, honey, granulated sugarcane juice, turbinado sugar, pure maple syrup, rice syrup, barley malt syrup and other forms of sugar except two. These two are blackstrap molasses, which is a good source of iron, and fructose (or fruit sugar), which is helpful to diabetics because it doesn't require insulin to get into the liver and body cells, so blood sugar levels remain fairly stable after eating it.

Though some advertisements might tout one or another type of sugar as more healthful than white table sugar, the truth is there's no nutritional advantage of one type of sugar over another, save for blackstrap molasses. Honey, for instance, contains minute amounts of minerals, but they are in such small quantities that they contribute no nutrients to the diet.

Because sugar contains calories and little else, it's considered an "empty" food and is best eaten in moderation. Sugar causes tooth decay and can play a role in obesity. It may also suppress the immune system and have other effects on the body not yet understood by scientists.

The main point: Recognize that sugar has little if any nutritional value and don't be fooled into believing that any type of sugar is good for you.

skills are a must. Without resorting to name-calling or using ridicule, you and your husband need to come to an understanding of what's best for your child. No single answer works for every family.

In some homes, meat is banished from the refrigerator, freezer and cupboards, and the meat eaters have their meaty meals at restaurants. Other homes permit meat inside its walls yet it's not given to the children—at least not while they're very young and show no interest in it. Still other homes allow the kids to freely eat vegetarian or meat-centered meals at home. You and your husband need to select the approach that works best for you.

Try to educate your husband in a nonthreatening manner about your vegetarian diet and why meatless eating is healthful for your child. When he understands that the vegetarian diet is not only healthful but also popular—with some twenty thousand American adults becoming vegetarian *each week,* studies show (no statistics are available for children)—he's bound to soften his attitude.

But even if your husband remains difficult, you *can* find support from vegetarian groups, which typically meet monthly for potlucks, holiday parties, recipe swapping and information. Hundreds of them operate in the United States and many more overseas. To find out the location and contact person for the vegetarian group nearest you, contact the Vegetarian Resource Group at (301) 366-VEGE. If there is no vegetarian group in your area, consider starting one. (See "Setting Up Your Own Veg Group," page 78.)

"My wife eats meat on occasion, and our three-year-old daughter has tasted it and likes it. We had agreed to raise her as a vegetarian; now she's siding with her mother."

T ry not to let dietary differences come between you and your wife or your daughter. You don't want to put your daughter in the position of choosing who's better, Mom or Dad, based on what you eat. No matter how strong you feel about the advantages of the vegetarian way of eating, avoid any holier-than-thou talk. Morals aren't the point. Personal healthful choices are.

You and your wife need to present a united front. In this case, it might be showing respect for one another's food choices. Your daughter needs to know what the family rules are. So sit down with your wife and talk, then communicate the rules clearly to your daughter.

Remember, though children like to wrap their parents around their little fingers, the grown-ups are still in charge.

SWEET SURRENDER

"My neighbor passes out Popsicles and cookies to her preschoolers and mine when they play together. How can I get her to provide more nutritious snacks—at least some of the time?"

A gain, communication is key. Though confronting someone, even in a pleasant manner, is difficult, you must speak up if the fact that your children regularly eat sweet snacks bothers you. You owe it to yourself to be honest with your feelings.

When speaking with your neighbor, appeal to her concern for the children's well-being. Gracefully tell her your stance on sweet snacks. Suggest healthful alternatives.

Then let the Popsicle sticks fall where they may. Your neighbor might take your concerns to heart and switch to fruit snacks, pretzels and other nutritious snacks immediately. Or she might hold firm and continue to hand out Popsicles and cookies. If she chooses the latter approach, you have decisions to make. One possibility is teaching your children to say no to sweet treats. This is easier said than done because preschoolers like to fit in with their peers—and, with few exceptions, they like sugar. Another possibility is inviting your preschoolers' friends to your house to play. In your domain, *you* have control over snack time. The last resort is to forbid your children to go to her friends' home.

Think hard before choosing this final route. In the world beyond your neighborhood, your preschoolers will have ample opportunities to eat sugary treats. Even bank tellers hand out lollipops. Then there are candy canes doled out by Santa, sweet treats shared at school parties and lemonade stands that cool the summer heat. You must decide which is worse: your children losing friends or letting them eat sugary snacks outside your home on occasion.

One thing's for sure: You can't change your neighbor if she refuses to change. But you can be a persuasive role model to your own kids.

FOOD ADDITIVES

"Some of the foods we eat come in boxes with long lists of ingredients including additives. Which additives should my family avoid?"

L et's break down food additives into two categories: questionable chemical additives and additives that might make some vegetarians squeamish.

In the first category, you'll find on product labels words like monosodium glutamate (MSG), mono- and diglycerides, calcium propionate and artificial flavorings and colors. Are these additives dangerous? Some are perfectly safe, others are questionable. It's impossible to know which is which unless you delve into the subject.

Some forty years ago, the U.S. Food and Drug Administration (FDA) developed a list of safe ingredients. Nicknamed GRAS for "generally recognized as safe," these ingredients included common ones such as salt as well as chemical additives.

The FDA continues ongoing investigations of additives. Yet some controversial additives make it on the GRAS list. MSG is one example. Some people who eat food containing MSG experience moderate reactions to it. For a complete GRAS listing, ask your librarian to help you locate the Code of Federal Regulations, Title 21, Part 170.

The Center for Science in the Public Interest, a consumer advocacy group based in Washington, D.C., says you ought to steer clear of some GRAS ingredients, like MSG. It also has a list of ingredients it considers detrimental to health. These ingredients include artificial food colorings (blue dyes no. 1 and no. 2, citrus red dye no. 2, green dye no. 3, red dye no. 3 and yellow dye no. 6), saccharin, sodium nitrate, butylated hydroxanisole (BHA), butylated hydroxtoluene (BHT), sulfur dioxide, sodium bisulfate and caffeine.

In the second category—the additives that make some vegetarians squeamish—rennet, casein and sugar top the list. Rennet, used in cheese making, comes from the lining of cows; it is a by-product of the beef industry. Casein, a hidden dairy product for vegans to avoid, is a milk protein that makes cheese melt. And sugar? It may be processed through a charcoal made from animal bones.

Knowing that, food additives can leave a bad taste in your mouth. But it's hard to cook from scratch every day when your schedule includes transporting kids to and from day care, working outside the home and dragging them to the supermarket. Just do your best to read labels and avoid the most harmful food additives as often as possible.

TEACHING VALUES

"We have cats and a dog at home, and our four-year-old son cares for them deeply. He even feeds them without my needing to remind him. When is a good time to start telling him about how meat production hurts animals?"

Now's the time for open discussion. As with any important topic—whether sex or animal factory farming—consider your child's ability to understand, and address your conversation to his level.

A good starting place is making the connection between animals and the neatly wrapped packages of meat at the supermarket. Tell him "beef" is cow, "pork" is pig, and "veal" is a baby calf. Remind him that chicken, turkey and fish—which go by their undisguised names—used to flap their wings and swim in the sea. Be truthful. Say that meat is the flesh of animals, but maintain a neutral tone. If you're inflammatory, your son may pick up your emotion but miss the information.

If you believe your child can stomach it, tell him about the cruelty that animals endure in animal factory farms. Remind him that the song "Old MacDonald's Farm" is not reality for nearly all farm animals. Nor are there any Auntie Ems counting chicks. Animal factory farming is pure economics—and it's frightening. Many people who enter a slaughterhouse never want to eat meat again. Even the Humane Society of the United States, considered a moderate voice in the animal welfare arena, objects to factory farming, which it calls abusive to animals. (For more on factory farming and animal welfare, see "Compassion for Animals," page 133.)

You won't want to share all of the gruesome details about animal factory farming with your young son. He'll be ready to hear more as he gets older. But when you say something simple like, "Mommy and Daddy don't eat meat because we care about animals, even chickens, cows and pigs," he'll start to get the message.

A NUTRITION QUIZ

Okay, okay—a chat on science can spell b-o-r-i-n-g. Eating is the fun part. And so are true-or-false quizzes. Here's a short quiz to help learn the basics of nutrition as painlessly as possible.

Most foods contain a mixture of the three major macronutrients in food—carbohydrates, protein, and fat. Most people tend to think protein is the most important, fat is a dirty word and carbohydrates are confusing. None of these beliefs are true.

Knowing about the three macronutrients will help you choose a healthful diet for your family. So sharpen a pencil and let's start.

TRUE OR FALSE:
Starches are fattening.

If you marked "false," award yourself 5 points. Starches, also known as complex carbohydrates, are a rightful mainstay of one's diet—whether or not you're trying to shed excess pounds. They are also rich in vitamins, minerals and fiber. Believe it or not, carbohydrates are the *only* food category not linked to any leading killer diseases.

Carbohydrates come in two types: starches (complex carbohydrates) and sugars (simple carbohydrates). Both types are made up of carbon, hydrogen and oxygen molecules. Starches look like branched chains, which digestive enzymes break down into sugars. These sugars are readily absorbed into the bloodstream and are used primarily for energy. Carbohydrates have four calories per gram, compared to a hefty nine calories in a single fat gram.

TRUE OR FALSE:
Consuming dietary fiber can prevent disease.

You get 5 more points if you said "true." Loading up on foods rich in fiber lowers your risk of colon cancer, diverticular disease (which affects the intestines), obesity, heart disease, diabetes, varicose veins and hemorrhoids, among other illnesses.

Fiber is an important nonnutrient, meaning it supplies no calories, vitamins or minerals to the body, but it keeps the digestive system running smoothly. Complex carbohydrates, which come from plants alone, are the only sources of fiber.

The recommended fiber intake for adults is twenty-five to thirty-five grams daily; the less food you eat, the less fiber you need, so most children need to eat fewer grams of fiber than adults. The best sources of fiber are complex carbohydrates, such as grains, vegetables, fruits and legumes. Skip dietary fiber supplements unless they're prescribed by a doctor. Encourage lots of fluids. And if you or your child is unaccustomed to eating a higher-fiber diet, increase the intake of fiber gradually to avoid, ahem, odoriferous consequences.

Many animal proteins contain more fat than protein.

Score another 5 points if you picked "true." Foods rich in protein often pack a hefty amount of fat. In hard cheeses, such as cheddar, one-fourth of the calories are protein; the rest are fat. In whole milk, about 20 percent of the calories are protein and about half are fat. Meats, too, are mostly fat. The calories in a steak are 20 percent protein and 80 percent fat. Chicken fares better, with about 65 percent of calories from protein and the remainder from fat. But in all animal foods, about half of the fat is saturated; saturated fat remains the nastiest villain in deadly diseases like heart disease.

Vegetarian foods can be rich in protein, but the remaining calories are usually carbohydrate. For instance, the calories of most legumes are about 25 percent protein and 75 percent carbohydrate. Exceptions include nuts and seeds, which are fatty.

It's been said that Westerners would excrete the most expensive urine in the world if the nitrogen it contains were harvested. The nitrogen comes from the excess protein Americans and other Westerners consume, both meat eaters and vegetarians. The building blocks of protein, called amino acids, are nitrogen-containing chemicals that are strung together to form long chains.

These proteins are used by the body for myriad functions: building and repairing tissues, transporting nutrients and oxygen in the body, aiding the clotting of blood, to name a few. Excluding water, about 50 percent of the body's weight is protein. Though it is vital, protein—especially animal protein—has been overplayed. As long as you eat a variety of foods and adequate calories, you'll get enough protein. (For more on protein, see "Protein—How Much for Good Health?" page 16.)

TRUE OR FALSE:
The average person's need for fat is four tablespoons a day.

Did you say "false"? If so, score 5 more points. Your actual daily need is only a mere tablespoon of fat to maintain good nutrition. You can get this fat without slathering your bread with butter. Some fat comes from foods, even vegetables and legumes, and some is added during cooking.

Though fat is necessary for good health, it's obviously overeaten. In fact, even though Americans are eating fewer calories than in the early 1900s, they are fatter due to an increase in inactivity and a greater consumption of fatty foods. About one in three Americans is overweight.

Unlike carbohydrates and proteins, dietary fat is believed to slip easily into body fat stores because it's in a form closely resembling body fat. Consider this: The Chinese consume about 20 percent more calories than Americans do, but aren't as heavy for their height, according to findings of the China Project, a massive epidemiological study. One reason is activity level; another is fat intake. The Chinese, on average, take in only 15 percent of total calories from fat. Americans eat more than double that amount. Other studies echo the China findings.

The good news is Americans are beginning to eat less fatty diets. According to the latest government nutrition survey, the average fat intake is 34 percent of calories. A decade ago, the average was 40 percent. That's an improvement, for sure, but we're not home free. Fat is still a heavyweight in the Western diet—and it's knocking out victims left and right.

Tally up your score: 20 points, nutrition champ; 10 or 15 points, in training; 5 points, go back to basics; 0 points, see a nutritionally aware doctor or other health professional.

SETTING UP YOUR OWN VEG GROUP

When you feel alone and are struggling with questions about raising your child as a vegetarian, you need support. If you can't find a vegetarian group in your area, consider starting one.

First, you'll need to find potential members. Post notices at local natural food stores, ethnic groceries and other food stores. Also send press releases to your town's newspaper. Or place an ad announcing your new group and when and where the first meeting will be.

Schedule the first meeting at someone's home, preferably your own, or at a church that agrees to donate space for your first meeting.

(Some churches or other meeting places charge a nominal fee.) At the meeting, find out why people have come, whether they have children and what their interests are.

Be sure to compile a list of everyone's name, address and phone number. Ask them to add the names of any friends or family members who might be interested in attending future meetings. At your first meeting, let everyone know the location and time of the second meeting. Consider making the second or third meeting a potluck, in which each person who attends brings a dish to pass. Potlucks offer a fun way for members to get to know one another.

Other possibilities for your veg group, depending on the interests of the members, are a monthly or quarterly newsletter, recipe swapping, family outings and meetings at restaurants that serve vegetarian food.

Your most important discovery will be that you're not alone. Other vegetarians with children need support too. You can lend each other a helping hand and share words of encouragement.

5

Your Grade-Schooler

When your child enters school, she goes through a lot of changes. She becomes more concerned with what her friends say than with what you think. Peer pressure is a reality—and some vegetarian kids want to eat meat to fit in. They need to belong. You can help your grade-schooler by encouraging her to join clubs and other activities that foster a sense of belonging. Though your child may love you deeply, she'll probably act cooler toward you, especially in the presence of other kids. But she still needs her family—and she knows it.

When you make new rules, such as junking the junk food or becoming vegetarian, your grade-schooler will probably balk. She has favorite foods and a desire for greater independence. This combo makes it difficult for a family to become vegetarian overnight. Yet you can make improvements to the family's meals gradually. Grade-schoolers want recognition as individuals, so appeal to your child's sense of responsibility—and to her taste buds. Also help her be sociable by letting her hang out with her friends and do the things they do, within reason, of course.

As long as you provide delicious food and are sensitive to your grade-schooler's need to belong and to become more independent, she'll like being vegetarian.

FAMILIES IN TRANSITION

"I stopped eating meat a few years ago to improve my health. The more I read, the more I realize that my kids need to eat better too. How can I improve my kids' diet without a revolt?"

Your dilemma mirrors the difficulty that hounded a family of eleven (a mom, a dad and nine kids). After the mom had her children, she decided to go vegetarian. Her eldest joined her right away. But how could she get her other eight children on board?

Here are some of her tips, along with other ideas from families in transition.

❖ Introduce tasty vegetarian meals to the family—with the emphasis on tasty. If your family usually eats meat at dinner, go vegetarian every other evening, increasing the number of vegetarian meals over time. Good bets are pasta, breakfast foods (even for dinner!), pizza with vegetable toppings, soup and salad, bean burritos and vegetable kebabs with rice.

❖ When you do serve meat, deemphasize it. For instance, if chili is on tonight's menu, load it up with legumes and vegetables and add only a smidgeon of beef. When making a chicken and vegetable stir-fry, go heavy on the vegetables and light on the chicken. Gradually reduce the amount of meat until it disappears altogether. The kids may not even notice.

❖ Avoid the cheese-and-egg pitfall. Some new vegetarians rely heavily on dairy products to replace the meat they've dropped from their diets. This is a nutrition no-no. Dairy products drip with fat and cholesterol, and they have no fiber. Buying the slimmed-down versions takes care of the fat problem only. For this reason, use cheese sparingly to give a bit of flavor. Eat cholesterol-laden eggs only in dishes where they are used as binders and leaveners (such as casseroles and quick breads). Resist frying up a plate of scrambled eggs.

❖ Try fake meats. Because most kids are creatures of habit, they may want an occasional burger or hot dog. Fortunately, in natural food stores and well-stocked supermarkets, you can find meat look- and

taste-alikes. Many of them are made primarily from soy. One caveat: Though fake meats are rich in complex carbohydrates and
contain no cholesterol, sometimes they are high in fat. Check
product labels. Some brands taste "meatier" than other brands, so
try different products to discover the ones your children like best.

❖ Experiment with textured vegetable protein. Made from soy and
sometimes wheat, textured vegetable protein (or TVP, for short, a
registered trademark of the Archer-Daniels-Midland Company) is
a wonderful replacement for ground beef. It tastes best in recipes
in which ground beef is one of many ingredients; sloppy joes and
tacos are two examples. TVP doesn't work well alone. So sauce it
up and enjoy.

❖ Serve up tofu and other quintessentially vegetarian foods when
the timing is right. Once your kids learn to enjoy some familiar
meatless meals, introduce foods they've never met: tofu, tempeh,
soy milk, uncommon grains like couscous and even sea vegetables.
Just don't get overzealous and place a platter of tempeh burgers
on the table expecting the family to dig in with gusto. A *gradual*
introduction is key. For instance, sauté cubes of tofu and add them
to a stir-fry, allowing your kids to pick them out if they don't like
them. Or "sneak" tofu into foods. The tofu in tofu-pumpkin pie
or in dips is barely noticeable.

❖ Allow your kids to eat meat occasionally. If they have a craving
for their favorite fast-food burger, let them indulge, knowing that
their day-to-day diet is nutritious. If you ban meat completely,
they might want it even more intensely.

❖ Give your testimony. Clearly state why you are vegetarian and
why you want your children to eat meatless meals. You're a persuasive role model. Use your influence to get them off to a healthful start. You can make a bigger difference than you might realize.

IT'S SOY GOOD

Lower your cholesterol. Fight cancer. Slow bone loss. Sound too good
to be true? Amazingly, dozens of studies, including an overview in
the *New England Journal of Medicine*, point to the humble soybean as

one answer to these health problems, elevating it to princely status in the nutrition kingdom.

It appears that soy protein can dramatically lower blood cholesterol levels—and that's great news for anyone with a family history of heart disease—as well as cut the risk of many forms of cancer and retard osteoporosis, a bone-thinning disease that affects many older women.

Though scientists don't completely understand how soy protein works its magic, they have some clues. Soy contains various substances like phytoestrogens, isoflavones and genistein, all of which play a role in inhibiting the formation of cancer cells. Genistein may also block several enzymes that tumor cells need to thrive and grow, so in effect the tumors are starved. Soy, by the way, is the only known source of genistein.

Also in favor of soy are epidemiological studies showing that heart disease and cancer are far less prevalent in countries, such as Japan, where soy foods remain staples. More specific are studies, such as one conducted at the University of Milan in Italy, in which patients already eating a low-fat diet experienced significant drops in "bad" cholesterol, or low-density lipoproteins, when soy protein was added to their diet. In only three weeks, their "bad" cholesterol plummeted an average of 21 percent. Other studies have found similar results.

While scientists make further discoveries, take advantage of the knowledge to date by serving soy foods to your family. And you won't have to overdose on tofu and its soy food cousins to get health benefits, nutrition experts say. One serving a day—a glass of soy milk or half a cup of tofu, for instance—may provide enough genistein to lower the risk of some cancers by half. Eating twice that much, or about twenty-five grams of soy protein, could improve cholesterol levels.

Here's a glance at the most common soy foods. If you can't find them at your supermarket, you'll need to visit your local natural food store or Asian market.

Soybeans. These small, cream-colored beans pack a nutritional punch. A 3 ½-ounce serving of cooked soybeans has 11 grams of protein and 4.5 grams of fiber. They have no cholesterol—that's true of all plant foods—and next to no saturated fat. For cooking instructions, see "Legume Cookery," page 174.

Soy flour. Made by grinding whole, dry soybeans, soy flour can improve the nutritional profile of muffins, pancakes, quick breads and other baked goods. Substitute soy flour for up to one-third of the wheat flour in your recipe. Don't use soy flour in yeasted breads because it lacks the gluten needed for rising. Store soy flour in an airtight container in your refrigerator to prevent rancidity.

Soy oil. Extracted from soybeans, soy oil contains linolenic acid, which may help prevent heart disease and cancer. It is one of the few plant sources of omega-3 fatty acids.

Soy milk. This tasty beverage is made by blending soaked soybeans with water, straining out the pulp and then cooking and cooling the remaining liquid. Commercial soy milks come in various flavors, including plain, almond and cocoa.

Soy yogurt. Cultured from soy milk using active bacteria cultures, this dairy-free treat is available in many flavors.

Tofu. The best-known soy food in America, tofu is the precipitated protein component of soy milk. Remember Little Miss Muffet who ate her curds and whey? Tofu is curd, which is pressed into blocks. Though this definition sounds unappealing, tofu can taste absolutely delicious, depending on how it's prepared. Some people like it straight out of the carton, but most prefer it incorporated in dishes.

Soft tofu, which contains more water than firm tofu, makes creamy dips, desserts and dressings. Firm and extra-firm tofu is best for cubing and slicing and works well in stir-fries and other dishes where you want the tofu to hold its shape.

Tofu is also available in seasoned and herbed varieties. It comes in "light" versions too, in which the fat content has been reduced by removing some of the oil in soy milk before it's turned into tofu.

Tempeh. Pronounced "*tem*-pay," this soy food is fermented soybean cakes. It has a pungent flavor that grows stronger with age. That's why most kids prefer fresh tempeh, which is relatively mild. If the tempeh has a few gray or black spots, it's still fine to eat. But when it develops a strong ammonia odor, toss it in the garbage. Tempeh may be marinated, steamed, grilled or sautéed. It works well in main-dish salads and many entrées.

Textured vegetable protein. The name may sound unpalatable—no wonder it's usually called TVP, a registered trademark of the Archer-Daniels-Midland Company—but the food tastes great in saucy dishes like spaghetti with tomato sauce, chili and sloppy joes. TVP is made from uncooked soybeans that have had their fat removed. The result is defatted soy flakes that may be reconstituted with water and used like ground beef. You can buy it in granule and chunky forms.

Miso. This traditional Japanese condiment is a salty paste made from cooked, aged soybeans. The darker the miso, the stronger the flavor. It makes a great base for soups and can flavor sauces, marinades and dips.

For more on soy foods, check out the health and cookbook sections in your local bookstore or library. One recommendation: Mark and Virginia Messina's *The Simple Soybean and Your Health* (Avery Publishing, 1994).

KID PLEASERS

"My second grader likes bean burritos, but her older brothers won't touch them. They prefer veggie burgers or pizza. I'm trying to please everyone by cooking several dinners each night, but I feel like a waitress."

No parent ought to be a short-order cook. But children shouldn't be forced to eat food they detest. Compromise is the ticket to hassle-free mealtimes.

When planning meals, select main dishes that all family members accept. If you're particularly energetic, plan two main dishes for some meals, saving any leftovers for quick dinners later in the week. Round out the evening's offerings with one or two side dishes that not only complement the main dish but also introduce a new food now and then. Encourage your children to try each dish. Many families have had success with the "no thank you" bite, in which children must eat one bite of each food but they are not forced to eat more of it.

Involve your children in the planning and cooking of meals. When your children participate in mealtime, they're more likely to eat their creations. Grade-schoolers can make salads, thread skewers for kebabs, slice fruit and complete other cooking tasks with some supervision.

When a child refuses to eat, consider his motivations. If he's ill, tuck him into bed and give him fluids to drink—or whatever the doctor orders. If his tummy's full, put a moratorium on after-school snacks. If he's just being plain ornery, excuse him from the table. You don't have to put up with his whining. But save his dinner. When he gets hungry later in the evening, he can finish it. Don't bow to any demands for a different meal. When you're consistent, he'll get the message loud and clear.

Show respect to your children and expect it in return. That means providing them good foods to eat, but not becoming their slave.

"My first grader gobbles up tofu. Her older brother refuses to try it or any other food he deems weird. Then he fills up on dessert."

Three thoughts come to mind. First, explain to your older child what the new food is. Then it won't seem so odd. Second, don't force him to eat it if he truly doesn't want it after trying a bite. Serve another nutritious food he likes. And, lastly, make dessert a healthful part of the meal. Sliced fruit is fine. Devil's food cake? Well, you know the answer.

If you permit your son to fill up on dessert without requiring him to eat dinner, you reward his unwanted behavior. His behavior will continue until you put a stop to it. When you don't know what to do, go back to basics: Offer a variety of delicious and nutritious foods, including a healthful dessert—and don't worry. Hungry kids invariably get enough variety and calories.

EATING AT FRIENDS' HOMES

"Our fifth-grade son asked a classmate to our home for dinner and wants me to cook meat for the boy. I've reassured our son that I'll make a dish everyone will like, but he's still worried."

In support of your family's vegetarian choice, don't cave into your son's request for a meat dish for his friend. There are ample meat-less meals that are well liked by almost everyone. Discuss the options with your son.

Then let him take charge. Ask him to select the menu, and as long as it's not outrageous, go along with his wishes. Your son will be pleased, and so will his friend. And your son is likely to feel more confident about the acceptability of the vegetarian diet. It's a win-win situation.

"My third grader has been invited to dinner at her best friend's home. The friend knows my daughter is a vegetarian, but they're afraid to tell the mother. Should I call?"

Age plays a big factor in this decision. If your daughter and her friend were teenagers, one of them ought to tell the mother. But the kids are young.

Your daughter might be frightened to make a special request, and her friend may not know how to explain your daughter's vegetarian choice. Talking to the mother yourself is a reasonable solution. You'll have an opportunity to thank the mother for her hospitality and to speak up about the healthfulness of the vegetarian diet. The mother is likely to listen and oblige without hesitation. Just have a few menu ideas up your sleeve in case the mother asks for suggestions.

Fast Food

"Our boy hangs out at fast-food restaurants with his friends and uses his weekly allowance to buy burgers and fries. Should we stop giving him his allowance?"

This is one of those apples-and-oranges questions. The purpose of an allowance is to teach your kid how to handle money properly. If you no longer give him an allowance, how can he learn how to save and spend? However, as his parents, you make rules concerning his allowance. That's perfectly fine. Some parents might forbid spending money on candy; you might outlaw burgers and fries.

Use this clash over money to your advantage. Talk to him about saving and spending and encourage him to make wise choices with his allowance. Your own saving and spending habits will influence him, of course. At the same time, recognize his need to be one of the gang. Letting him hang out with friends, dress, talk and goof off with them and have the same privileges as they do helps him be sociable and get along with others.

In deciding how to handle the burger-and-fries situation, weigh his need to be sociable versus his diet. Remember, if he's been vegetarian for all or most of his life, it's likely he'll return to his vegetarian beginnings. (See "Fitting In," page 102.)

Also consider acceptable ways he might fit in with his peers. Suggest to him that he might frequent fast-food restaurants that have vegetarian options. Don't even mention the name "McDonald's"— the only veg food it sells is salad, and few guys are going to order a salad. Very uncool. Instead, think of places where veg food is inconspicuous: a bean burrito at a taco joint or mushroom pizza at a pizza place. If your son says, "Hey, let's go get some pizza," before anyone pushes for burger town, he'll have vegetarian options.

Another possibility is his joining a sports team, club, school band or a church youth group, where he'll receive the sense of belonging and acceptance he needs from his peers. He will still run into tough choices, such as when the team stops at a hot dog stand on their way home from a game. You, too, have encountered many sticky situations. Let him know how you've handled them. Your experience can help.

As you brainstorm ideas with your son, be sure to let him know the valued place he has in your family. Right now, during his school years, he needs to know he belongs.

AN OVERNIGHT VEGETARIAN

"My sixth grader announced to the family that she's a vegetarian and will no longer eat the meals I make. I'm confused and worried about her health."

So the tables have turned. Your little one—who's not so little anymore—is asserting herself and insisting on meatless meals. Be reassured: A child stepping out on her own is a sign of blossoming maturity, and she selected a healthful way to come into her own.

That said, know that a healthful vegetarian diet leads to a long life and prevents disease. It also provides ample protein, iron, calcium and other nutrients. Just browse the various questions and answers throughout these chapters and you'll learn for yourself how health-supporting the vegetarian diet is. Keep in mind that a healthful vegetarian diet has the solid backing of the American Dietetic Association and the American Academy of Pediatrics.

But not all self-designed vegetarian diets are healthful. If left to their own devices, some kids would become junk-food vegetarians. Their menus would be nightmares: sugary cereals, potato chips, french fries, candy bars, doughnuts, grilled cheese sandwiches and soda pop. (Curiously, this diet mimics that of many meat-eating kids, except that they also wolf down burgers loaded with fat and cholesterol.)

Because some new vegetarian kids might make poor food choices, you need to provide guidance. Encourage your grade-schooler to eat whole grains, vegetables, fruits and legumes and to limit her consumption of fats and sweets. Dairy products and eggs are optional. (See "Becoming a Vegan," page 112.)

Try your best to see your daughter's new dietary choice as positive, but don't be surprised if you might view it as a rejection of family values. In their book *The New Vegetarians*, psychologists Paul R. Amato and Sonia A. Partridge write, "Some parents are upset by what they

Trick or Treat?

Halloween is tricky for health-minded families who want to treat kids to true goodies. Though a once-a-year gorge won't have lasting health effects, why encourage eating candy until your kids are moaning with stomachaches? Here are ideas for a truly happy Halloween.

❖ Ration candy. Allow your children several pieces of candy on Halloween, then dole out only one or two pieces a day thereafter. Parents who ration candy often discover that the kids forget about their stashes in a week or so.

❖ Opt for a hard-love approach. On Halloween, go along with your kids' fiendish desire to eat gobs of candy, knowing full well they'll feel sick to their stomachs. Then, while they're experiencing discomfort, inform them in a friendly tone of voice that overeating candy causes stomachaches. When another holiday rolls around, remind them how sick they felt on Halloween. Your kids will think twice before overindulging in sweets.

❖ Buy your kids' Halloween candy from them. That's right. Give them a few pennies for each piece of candy—or a dollar or two for the lot. Then trash the candy. If you're concerned about wasting food—assuming candy could be considered real food—remember that eating empty calories is also a waste.

perceive as the 'radicalization' of their children. They had wanted nice normal children, but they got vegetarians instead.

"Given time to adjust," they continue, "many parents find that occasionally preparing vegetarian food for their children is not as difficult as they had thought. Many realize for the first time that meatless meals can be satisfying and delicious. Some even come to enjoy the challenge, and novelty, of cooking vegetarian food."

Amato and Partridge found that 66 percent of parents and other family members were initially opposed to their children's dietary change, 16 percent were indifferent, 10 percent were supportive and 8 percent had mixed reactions.

❖ Throw a Halloween party in which the treats are apples, oatmeal cookies, pumpkin muffins and other true goodies. The kids could wear their costumes, carve pumpkins under adult supervision and play games, such as bobbing for apples and "bat, bat, spider" (use the same rules as "duck, duck, goose"). Be sure to get your neighbors or friends involved.

❖ Forbid trick-or-treating, but don't count on winning the parent-of-the-year award. A less drastic measure is to inspect your kids' hauls, sorting the stuff into acceptable and unacceptable piles. Sugarless gum, boxes of raisins, coins and stickers go in the acceptable pile and everything else in the no-good pile. (Again, expect no rewards.)

❖ When you give out treats to little goblins, make them wholesome: small toys such as spider rings, sparkly pencils, stickers and coins. If you prefer to make your own homemade goodies, be sure to securely attach a tag with your name, address and phone number, and hand them out only to children whose parents you know. Otherwise, your well-intentioned treats may end up in their trash.

Next to Christmas, Halloween is most kids' favorite day of the year. The trick is making it healthful.

When a child becomes a vegetarian, changes in family relationships invariably follow. Some relationships weaken, but others grow closer and stronger. That's right: Stronger family relationships are one more potential benefit of the vegetarian diet.

TEASING

"Since I'm a vegetarian and my wife is not, we've decided to let our kids choose the way they want to eat. The problem is our eldest son, who has turned into a holier-than-thou vegetarian. He teases his little brothers about 'murdering chickens.'"

When some family members are vegetarians and others eat meat, food fights can erupt at the dinner table. What's most important is how they are handled.

The childhood rhyme "Sticks and stones may break my bones, but names can never hurt me" is a lie. Words can hurt. They can insult, ridicule, belittle and shame. Name-calling and hurtful words have no legitimate place in a warm home.

You might want to meet privately with your son and remind him that teasing can hurt others, even if meant in jest. At the same time, commend him on his commitment to his vegetarian diet. When you point out that the vegetarian diet celebrates life (personal health, the environment and animals), he might see that hurtful words have no place in your home, where you've upheld the value of differences.

Then consider having a family meeting in which you and your wife express that each family member has a right to make his or her own food choices—within reason. You wouldn't want your children to believe they have a "right" to eat Oreo cookies for dinner. Make it clear that you won't tolerate name-calling and hurtful words. This problem might pop up again, with your youngest teasing your eldest about being a cabbage head. Good luck.

"Children in my second grader's class tease him for being a vegetarian. I know he's bothered though he won't admit it. How can I help my son?"

First, keep communication lines open so that your son feels he can turn to you when he's troubled. In their highly acclaimed book *How to Talk So Kids Will Listen & Listen So Kids Will Talk*, authors Adele Faber and Elaine Mazlish say parents can help by acknowledging their children's feelings and listening with full attention. It is also important to ask open-ended questions or make statements that show you see something is wrong. A simple example is, "You look sad."

Also talk to him about teasing in general, making it clear that teasing is bad if it hurts people. Your son needs to hear this message if he thinks he's odd because he's a vegetarian. He might think he's at fault for his classmates' inappropriate behavior.

Help him feel one of the gang too. When your son has friends over for lunch or a birthday party, serve favorite kid foods like pizza or spaghetti. Save the lentil-nut loaf for family night.

Another possibility is to speak to your son's class about the vegetarian diet once you have the teacher's okay. Be sure to bring in tasty and wholesome samples, such as carrot-raisin muffins or English muffin pizzas, to help show that eating vegetarian foods is a delicious choice. Before you contact the teacher, make sure your son is comfortable with this idea.

Finally, consider joining a vegetarian group in your area. Many of them have family potlucks and picnics, where your son can meet other vegetarian kids. He'll learn that he's not alone.

SCHOOL LUNCHES

"The hot lunches at school are horrendous, so I pack lunches for my kids. But they feel funny that they have healthful lunches while their friends fill up on fried foods and junk."

You're right on the money about lunches served in school cafeterias. Averaging 38 percent of calories from fat (compared to the oft-repeated goal of 30 percent), 15 percent of fat calories from saturated fat (the desired amount is no more than 10 percent) and fifteen hundred milligrams of sodium (the target is eight hundred milligrams), these lunches set up kids for serious illness later in life.

Studies have shown that kids eating the standard American diet, which mirrors today's school lunch, demonstrate a strong link between their blood cholesterol levels and lesions in their arteries. In one ten-year study by researchers at Louisiana State University, the children who had the highest levels of total blood cholesterol and low-density lipoproteins (or LDL, the "bad" cholesterol) had the most fatty streaks in their arteries. Those with the highest levels of high-density lipoproteins (or HDL, the "good" cholesterol) had the fewest fatty streaks.

The obvious conclusion: Kids need to eat less saturated fat. Schools aren't going to lead the charge toward more healthful lunches. With the need to make their lunches affordable, schools rely heavily on surplus commodities from the U.S. Department of Agriculture (USDA), primarily whole milk, butter, ground pork and ground meat (all of which drip with saturated fat).

Also saddling the schools are rules required by the National

Packing a School Lunch

Kids' lunches can become a battle of wills because children want what other kids have—and often the popular goodies aren't good for health. Here are some yummy ideas.

❖ Peanut butter and jelly sandwich with a twist. Instead of fatty peanut butter on bread, mix together equal parts of peanut butter and part-skim ricotta cheese or reduced-fat soft tofu. Spread this mixture and fruit preserves on whole-wheat bread.

❖ PLT sandwich, with the "P" standing for pickles. Between slices of whole-grain bread, place pickles (sweet or dill), lettuce and tomato plus favorite condiments.

❖ Cheese and vegetable sandwich. The key is slicing the cheese very thin so the sandwich isn't fat-filled. Place the cheese on whole-grain bread with favorite vegetables: cucumber and tomato slices, olives, shredded carrot and/or zucchini rounds.

❖ Tahini and banana sandwich. Tahini is a thick paste of raw sesame seeds. It tastes great spread on whole-wheat bread and topped with slices of banana.

❖ Say "yo" to yogurt. Spoon 8 ounces of nonfat plain yogurt into a sealable container. Stir in ½ to 1 cup of sliced fruit, seal the container and freeze. In the morning, pack it in your child's lunch box. By lunchtime, the yogurt will no longer be frozen but will still be cool enough to enjoy. Don't forget a spoon.

❖ Baked tortilla chips. These have flavor and crunch but little or no fat. An ideal alternative to potato chips.

❖ Fresh fruits or small cans of fruit packed in their own juices. Buy the kind with pull-tops.

❖ Mini rice cakes in various flavors, including honey nut.

❖ Air-popped popcorn. Pack the popcorn in zipper-type bags to keep it fresh.

❖ Low-fat and fat-free cookies. Make your own or buy commercial varieties of your kids' favorites. Some are sweetened with fruit juices rather than refined sugar. Check product labels.

School Lunch Program, which feeds about 30 million children every day. The rules include a specific amount of meat or "meat alternate," two or more vegetables and/or fruits, a bread or "bread alternate" and milk. Even the USDA criticized the school lunch program for not meeting federal nutrition guidelines in its own evaluation, prompting Senator Patrick Leahy, a Democrat from Vermont, to propose a sweeping reform of the program. Clearly, with the USDA's requirement of meat, there is a built-in prejudice against the vegetarian diet.

Yet you can provide nutritious lunches to your kids. The best ones are low in fat, sodium and sugar and rich in nutrients. But they also must be delicious and acceptable in your children's eyes and in the view of their classmates. If their friends laugh at their lunches, then into the trash they may go.

It's smarter to send them to school with PB&J on whole-wheat bread and a piece of fruit than to pack a lunch of tofu cubes and sprouts stuffed into pita bread. The first lunch is "normal"; the second lunch is "weird."

Being sensitive to your child's needs to fit in with his peers, check out more lunch suggestions in "Packing a School Lunch," page 94.

If you are really interested in improving school lunches, you might follow in the footsteps of Gail Heebner and Mary Hand-Mauser. Both of these women worked with their children's schools to offer nutritious lunches that meet government regulations and that kids like. Heebner managed to convince 201 public schools in the Raleigh, North Carolina, area to serve vegetarian meals for the Great American Meatout, a day set aside each year to encourage people across the nation to eat a meatless diet. She has continued to work with schools to improve lunch options. Hand-Mauser presented her children's parochial school in Louisville, Kentucky, with ideas for a pilot lunch program and managed to get a grant to help pay for healthful foods. She even achieved her goal to have a daily vegetarian option.

Whether you make a difference on a large scale or just in your own kitchen, you're doing your kids a big favor. The earlier you start, the better. By the time kids reach their teens, they've grown accustomed to the taste of fatty, salty and sweet foods and resist change. So start now—if you haven't already.

DIFFERENT RULES AFTER DIVORCE

"When my children spend the weekend at my ex-husband's home, he serves them meat and lets them eat as much junk food as they want. I've tried to discuss this matter with him, asking him to show greater care in choosing foods, but he won't listen."

D ivorce is difficult in so many ways. Food differences seem inconsequential compared to the greater pains of a family breakup. However, the problem is real. You want the best for your children, including their diet. Your ex doesn't share your concern about eating good food. Or maybe he's trying to win the kids' affection by giving them treats. In either case, your frustration with your ex is understandable. You may even have wondered whether he is trying to get back at you through them.

As you know, you can't change another person. You can change only yourself. Since your attempts at influencing your ex haven't worked, you could try talking with your children about food. Give them reasons to turn down meat and junk food. Encourage them to ask for meatless meals (spaghetti with tomato sauce and cheese pizza are two examples) and for fruit as snacks when they're with their father.

If your kids start eating less junk food when they're with your ex, great. If not, be confident in knowing that you are feeding them well. But let them know that no matter what they do or what they eat, you'll love them. They need your support in every way during this difficult time.

ORGANIC FOODS—ARE THEY REALLY BETTER?

Choosing organically grown foods, which by definition aren't treated with pesticides and other "cides," has the obvious health advantage of reducing your family's consumption of chemical residues. Now you have another reason to go organic: Organic produce may be richer in nutrients.

A scientific comparison of organic and conventional apples, pears, potatoes, corn and wheat found that the organic produce contained, on average, 63 percent more calcium, 59 percent more iron and 60 percent more zinc than conventional produce. Overall, the organic produce contained more than twenty out of twenty-two trace minerals studied. The study also found that organic produce had lesser amounts, on average, of several harmful substances, including 40 percent less aluminum, 29 percent less lead and 25 percent less mercury.

Selecting organic foods sends another message: that you value this earth. Overwhelming research shows that pesticide use damages soil, pollutes the environment (air, water and land) and endangers our food supply because pests develop a tolerance to the chemicals sprayed on produce and are harder to kill, setting the stage for crop devastation. That's just a taste of the harm that chemicals can cause to the earth, not to mention the workers, often poor immigrants, who handle them.

An increasing number of farsighted scientists support sustainable agriculture. Using techniques like crop rotation and the introduction of crop-friendly bugs that scare off plant-munching insects, farmers can avoid chemicals and save a bundle of money in the long run. Sustainable agriculture isn't new. In fact, it's very old, stretching back to our ancestors, who knew nothing of insecticides, fungicides and the other "cides."

You, too, can have an influence. By purchasing organic produce, you vote for the earth with your dollars—and money speaks.

When you buy organic produce, shop wisely. Look for food that's *certified* organically grown. Only a handful of states have certification, which indicates the food is free of pesticides and other chemicals. Fortunately, California, which supplies loads of produce to other parts of the nation, is among the states with certification. If the produce isn't clearly marked, ask the store manager whether the organic produce is certified.

When buying conventional produce, steer clear of vegetables and fruits grown outside the United States. That's because chemical manufacturers, whose pesticides are illegal to use in the United States, sell these products to other countries, where they're sprayed on produce, which is then sent to the United States and sold in supermarkets. Dubbed "the circle of poison," this roundabout trip can sneak illegal pesticides onto your kids' dinner plates.

Your best bet is growing an organic garden. When you garden organically, you're guaranteed cheaper food that tastes better than the supermarket's offerings and is guaranteed chemical-free. (An exception is planting in soil treated with chemical fertilizers. To be on the safe side, have your soil tested.) In addition, a garden is a wonderful lesson for kids. Few children have spent time on a farm, so they disconnect the earth from the food they see in supermarkets. Watching plants grow and mature—and end up in a stir-fry or another family favorite—can bring home a vital point: The earth is among our most vital resources.

Organic gardening is easier than you might imagine. If you're a beginner, get a book or two from the library or your local bookstore to learn more about feeding the soil, dealing with weeds and ridding your garden of pests and diseases.

6

The Bridge Years

A s your preteen catapults into puberty, his need to belong becomes fierce. Belonging isn't only a matter of having cool
friends. It also encompasses the desire to feel okay among all his
peers, especially now as he experiences bodily changes.

No wonder this stage can be tough. Vegetarian preteens might
want to hide their dietary preference from their classmates or go
along with the fast-food crowd. With self-consciousness and touch-
iness as the hallmarks of this age group, your once carefree vegetarian
grade-schooler might become difficult as he heads into his tumultu-
ous teens.

Fortunately, the vegetarian diet has become cool in many preteen
and teen social circles. So your child might win popularity points
because he's vegetarian. Go figure.

MAKING THEIR OWN CHOICES

*"My family rarely eats meat at home, but when we eat out, our three kids usually
order meat dishes. So do my husband and I. Some of our vegetarian friends say we
should stop eating meat altogether. We'd rather take it slow."*

Y our vegetarian friends have good intentions—the vegetarian diet
is good for you and the planet—but what's fine for them may
not be fine for you and your children right now. Instead of criticism,

you ought to receive support in your path toward a meatless diet.

The truth is, when eaten infrequently or as a complement to a meal, meat can be part of an overall healthful diet. Consider the Mediterranean diet. It bursts with vegetables, fruits and grains and contains minimal amounts of fish, cheese and poultry. The people who eat such a diet on the Greek island of Crete have a 98 percent lower rate of heart disease deaths than that of Americans.

Surely, eating less meat makes health sense. But becoming a vegetarian overnight isn't appropriate for everyone. Though some seasoned vegetarians recommend the cold-turkey approach (please pardon the pun), others say the gradual approach is best. When going green slowly but surely, you and your family have time to adjust to your new way of eating.

There are three basic gradual approaches, all of which can work for a heavy meat eater or for a near vegetarian. One approach is to dump red meat first, then chicken and finally fish. Another approach allows you to continue eating chicken a la king and fish sticks—just less and less frequently. For instance, you might drop one or two meat meals from the week's menu the first week. Then omit another two or three meat meals the second week until you discover that you no longer eat any meat.

The final approach is to reduce the amount of meat eaten at any given meal, reaching the point where the meat has vanished. For instance, make your usual lasagna with half the amount of meat. Cut it in half again the next time you make lasagna, and so on.

Meanwhile, in a nondefensive tone, remind your vegetarian friends that everyone needs to find his or her way on the vegetarian path. If your family is comfortable with eating meat occasionally, then follow your gut instincts. At the same time, be open to the possibility of making further dietary improvements.

In time, your vegetarian friends will accept you as you are and embrace your decision. It's who you are, not what you eat, that truly matters.

"A couple of weeks ago, my son announced that he's an environmentalist and a vegetarian. He fixes peanut butter and jelly sandwiches every night for dinner. I've tried to understand, but I don't."

When children refuse to eat the meals you've been serving for years, it's normal to react negatively. The squabbles come first, then the health worries, followed by a few lectures, and finally—if the parents remain open-minded—acceptance of the kid's new diet.

In the 1960s and '70s, when many young people became vegetarians, their reasons centered around politics and rebellion against the powers that be (in other words, anyone over thirty). In the 1980s, as study after study lauded the healthfulness of eating less meat and more grains, legumes, vegetables and fruit, Americans became more willing to accept the vegetarian diet. According to studies, about twenty thousand adult Americans joined the vegetarian ranks *each week* between the mid-eighties and the mid-nineties and continue to do so. Reliable numbers for kids don't exist, but indications—such as new publications for veg kids and the increasing number of kids' vegetarian groups—suggest that children are becoming vegetarians in sizable numbers too.

Not surprisingly, with today's emphasis on the health of the planet, many vegetarian children say they adopted their new diet because of environmental concerns. (For adults, the number-one reason is health, according to a survey by research firm Yankelovich, Clancy, Shulman, Inc.)

Meanwhile, you've got a problem: A son or daughter cannot live on peanut butter and jelly alone. The most open-minded parents would learn how to cook vegetarian meals and serve them to the family every evening. But that's not realistic. You need time to adjust to your son's decision to become a vegetarian. Eating is a universal language. When your son changed his diet, he changed the way the entire family communicates. You can't be expected to learn his new language at the snap of your fingers.

Yet parents with vegetarian children have learned new ways. They scour vegetarian cookbooks for family-pleasing recipes and start cooking vegetarian dinners a few times a week. When they make their standby recipes, such as spaghetti with meat sauce, they set aside a portion of the sauce before adding the meat. They also might put the child in charge of some of the cooking, easing pressure on the parents to cook a vegetarian meal or provide a meatless option at every dinner.

Typically, as a result of a family member becoming a vegetarian, the family's eating habits shift closer to a vegetarian diet. Sometimes siblings want to follow in the footsteps of their vegetarian brother or sister. Parents have made the switch too. And don't be surprised when your friends or family members say they're eating less meat too. The tables have turned. The vegetarian diet is "in."

FITTING IN

"I discourage my daughter from eating what her nonvegetarian friends eat just to fit in with her peers. But fitting in is so important when you're thirteen years old. I wonder if I should leave her alone."

There come those times in every parent's life when you're faced with the struggle of letting go. Letting go starts early, when you happily exchange your child's diapers for training pants. Later, the first day of kindergarten signals your need to give more space to your child in her school years. Now, in her junior high years, your not-so-little girl wants to be one of the gang.

Fitting in is important. The sense of belonging and acceptance shapes one's self-esteem. Your daughter might want to test the waters of meat eating. But if she's like many kids who've been vegetarian for all or most of their lives, she won't swim far. Social observers say that today's budding teenagers and their older brothers and sisters reflect their parents' values more often than we might think they do. So if you've held on to your vegetarian convictions, it's quite likely your daughter will too.

Interestingly, many of today's preteens and teens find out that their peers think the vegetarian diet is cool. It sets them apart. It shows that they have a mind of their own. Sure, they still might endure a few jokes now and then, and they might even eat meat occasionally.

But all in all, the lessons you taught your daughter about food in childhood will stick. If you demand that she not eat meat, she might rebel just to aggravate you. Give her some space and don't worry. Worry serves no good purpose.

Withstanding Peer Pressure

As kids enter their bridge years, they will face a fierce desire to be like their friends. If the grunge look is in—or bell-bottoms, who knows?—they'll want to wear the same clothes, talk the same way, do the same things and, quite possibly, eat the same foods as their peers do.

Many vegetarian sons and daughters stick to their healthful beginnings through these years; some do not. The question is, what should you do when your preteen shows a desire for meat? Here are some ideas.

- Do serve delicious vegetarian meals at home. Your example leaves a lasting impression on your child.
- Don't become overly strict with food. If you give your child a guilt trip when she admits to eating a burger and fries with her friends, you risk closing down communication lines. She might even eat meat to spite you.
- Do remind your child why your family is vegetarian. Hearing the reasons again—health, environmental, animal rights, spiritual and so on—might help her feel strong enough about her vegetarian convictions to stick with a meatless diet.
- Do give your child some examples of what she could say when she feels pressured to eat meat. For instance, these statements might trigger some ideas for her to use: "Meat isn't cool. It ruins our planet. And that stinks." Or "Hey, I'm not eating that stuff. I'm not ready to die yet." Or "Didn't you know Vanessa Williams (or k. d. lang or Natalie Merchant) is a vegetarian?"
- Don't cook meat for your child unless you really want to. When she sees you stick to your convictions, she may be encouraged to be equally strong among peers.
- Do help your child find support. There may be a vegetarian group or a pro-environment group in your area that she can join. She could also subscribe to vegetarian publications or surf the Internet for veg friends.

GROWTH SPURTS

"My eleven-year-old is growing by leaps and bounds. Will her vegetarian diet supply enough nutrition during her growth spurt?"

Most definitely. During the two years of rapid physical growth that precede a girl's first menstrual period, she will need more nutrients and calories. But here's the key: She will get her dietary needs met very easily because she will be eating more food. As she eats you "out of house and home," she'll be providing herself with vitamins, minerals, protein, carbohydrates and everything else she needs during her growth spurt.

Research shows that the meatless choice is perfectly healthful for girls and boys. One study easing vegetarian parents' concerns compared body measurements and nutrient intakes of ovo-lacto vegetarian kids aged ten to twelve (all of whom were vegetarian since birth) with meat-eating kids of the same age and socioeconomic class. All of the children were within or above the normal range for body size for their age group.

SPORTS AND NUTRITION

"Both of our children are very active in sports. What foods should they eat regularly to ensure that they're not shortchanged nutritionally?"

Foremost, they need a balanced diet. That means variety. When your children eat a varied diet—a mix of grains, legumes, vegetables and fruits, and dairy products and eggs if desired—they will get ample nutrients as long as they're eating enough calories.

Eating a balanced diet may sound easy, but anyone can fall into an unhealthful food rut. Consider this day's worth of meals: toast and jelly with milk for breakfast; a cheese sandwich and chips washed down with more milk for lunch; and lasagna, corn and garlic bread for dinner, followed by a fruit roll-up as a snack. Yes, these meals are meatless but they're lacking vegetables, fruits and legumes. Here's a solution: Replace the milk with fruit juice at breakfast, add an apple at lunch and a three-bean salad at dinner, and you have a more varied diet.

If your children eat no dairy products or eggs—only 4 percent of vegetarians are vegans (eating no animal products whatsoever)— they'll need vitamin B_{12}-fortified foods. Meeting the recommended dietary allowance for B_{12} is easy: A fortified breakfast cereal, fortified soy milk or a multivitamin can do the trick.

Another possible pitfall for vegetarian kids is eating too many dairy products. Some uninformed vegetarians rely heavily on dairy products to replace meat, but the sad result is a diet that's fatty and loaded with cholesterol. And fat, as you know, ought to be limited after a child reaches two years of age. In case you're concerned about protein or calcium intake, be reassured. A varied vegetarian diet supplies these nutrients abundantly. (See "Protein—How Much for Good Health?" page 16, and "Calcium Concerns," page 14.)

To round out a balanced diet, you need to junk the junk. Vegetarians in general eat less junk food than the average meat eater, but some subsist on junk food, which may not contain meat but is filled with other undesirables: fat, salt and sugar. It's best to limit them.

When your children eat a healthful vegetarian diet—which, by definition, has variety—they consume more nutrients than their meat-eating peers. In fact, a meat-centered diet is not balanced, being heavy on protein, fat and cholesterol and light on fiber. On a vegetarian diet, your kids will have an abundance of good food that will fuel them for their sports.

"Our eighth grader is on the soccer team and has started weight lifting to gain size and strength. He thinks he needs to eat meat for building muscle. Does he?"

R ocky Balboa had it all wrong when he slurped down raw eggs and feasted on meat to gain strength. Meat doesn't build muscle. Exercise does.

Studies show that the overwhelming majority of Americans eat two to three times the recommended dietary allowance for protein. Even vegetarians get more protein than their bodies need. (See "Protein—How Much for Good Health?" page 16.) Protein has very important functions, including repairing muscle tissue. But it's myth that meat is necessary for building muscle.

Veg Sports Heros

Here are some top athletes with one thing in common: a vegetarian diet, which they say gives them an edge in their sport.

Peter Burwash, Canadian Davis Cup tennis player
Andreas Cahling, medalist in the Mr. World bodybuilding competition
Chris Campbell, Olympic bronze medalist in wrestling
Gary Fanelli, winner of several marathons
Kathy Johnson, Olympic silver medalist in gymnastics
John McCarthy, professional baseball relief pitcher
Edwin Moses, Olympic gold medalist in the 400-meter hurdles
Martina Navratilova, tennis star
Bill Pearl, Mr. Universe, the premier men's bodybuilding award
Marjo Selin, finalist in the Ms. Olympia contest, the premier event in professional women's bodybuilding

---

Just take a look at bodybuilders Bill Pearl, Andreas Cahling and Marjo Selin. These three top athletes fuel their bodies with a vegetarian diet, heavy on carbohydrates. Complex carbohydrates, such as pasta, vegetables and legumes, are the body's best fuel. They provide energy in addition to nutrients. They are digested more quickly than high-protein, high-fat animal products. After eating a thick steak, most athletes feel sluggish—the opposite of the revved-up feeling they desire.

The upshot: Exercise will strengthen your son's muscles, and complex carbohydrates provide the fuel for his weight lifting and soccer. Contrary to popular belief, meat has no place on the training table.

ONSET OF MENSTRUATION

"My twelve-year-old girl just started having periods. Does she now need more iron in her diet?"

Menstruating girls and women do need a little extra iron in their diet because they lose some iron in their blood during menstruation and need to replenish their stores. The recommended dietary allowance (RDA) for iron in females eleven years to fifty years is fifteen milligrams, or five milligrams higher than for premenstrual girls or postmenopausal women. Remember, the RDAs are set high intentionally, so your daughter probably could safely eat a third less than the recommended amount, or about ten milligrams a day.

Suzanne Havala, a registered dietitian who wrote the American Dietetic Association's position papers on vegetarian diets, says that Western vegetarians are no more likely to court an iron deficiency than meat eaters. Yet it's possible for vegetarians (and meat eaters too) to have an iron deficiency. This occurs when not enough iron is absorbed from food to replace what is lost.

Before you panic, remember three things. First, anemia caused by iron deficiency doesn't happen overnight. In fact, acquiring an iron deficiency is a rather slow process. Second, meat is *not* required to avoid iron deficiency. Vegetarians who eat a healthful diet, including vitamin C, which aids in iron absorption, can have excellent blood levels of iron. (And, once the body absorbs iron, it handles this mineral in the same way whether it came from raisins or steak.) Third, getting enough iron isn't difficult.

Legumes, dried fruits, leafy green vegetables like spinach, and some grains contain very respectable amounts of iron. (See "Iron-Rich Foods," page 13.) Though the iron in plant foods is less absorbable than the iron in meat, you can make a significant difference by eating foods that aid iron absorption. Top on the list are foods containing vitamin C. As little as twenty-five milligrams of vitamin C— about one-quarter cup of orange juice—can nearly double your absorption of iron-containing plant foods.

The time to worry is when your daughter or any loved one feels tired, weak, irritable and downright crummy. These symptoms may point to an iron deficiency or other ailment. The only way to confirm an iron deficiency is through a blood test.

SLOW MATURATION

"I've read that some vegetarian children don't mature physically as soon as meat-eating children do. Should I be concerned?"

Studies have shown that girls on diets low in animal fats tend to have their first period several years later than girls eating diets rich in animal fats. For instance, in China, where the diet is primarily vegetarian and low in fat, the average age of the onset of menstruation is seventeen, ranging from fifteen to nineteen. Not only do these young women have a later period (according to Western standards) but also they enjoy far lower incidences of heart disease, cancer and obesity later in life. In rural Africa, girls also have their first period at about seventeen.

When girls switch from a low-fat, primarily vegetarian diet to a meat-centered diet, their first periods occur earlier. In Japan during the past forty years, the average age of menarche has dropped from 15.2 to 12.5 years. At the same time, the Japanese diet has become more similar to the average American diet.

What about the United States? The United States, as well as England, Norway, Denmark and other Western countries, has seen a downward creep of the onset of menstruation, according to the World Health Organization, which keeps statistics on the age of puberty. In 1840, when the vast majority of people ate a "peasant" diet, which contained far more grains and vegetable foods and far less meat than today's typical diet, the average girl had her first period at seventeen. Today the average is twelve and a half.

High-fat diets also cause early maturation in boys and an increase in incidence of baldness in men. But researchers don't have as many hard numbers on boys as on girls. This is simply because girls' maturation is easy to mark while boys' maturation isn't clear-cut.

The reason behind the differences in maturation is the effect of fat on hormone levels. Boys and girls—and men and women—who eat a meat-centered diet have more testosterone in their blood than do people on vegetarian or lower-fat diets. They also have more estrogen, studies show. So while hormones are affected by heredity, what a person eats also makes a difference.

Is later physical maturation in children a concern? By no means. Vegetarian girls may have slower breast development and get their periods later than their meat-eating peers. And vegetarian boys may experience a deepening of their voices and a broadening of their shoulders later than other boys. But vegetarian kids reach maturity just fine. There is no evidence that they endure any health problems due to later maturation. To the contrary, vegetarians are less likely than meat eaters to be victims of heart disease and other degenerative diseases, and they outlive meat eaters by several years.

POOR MODELS?

"We're vegetarians but I allow some snacks and ice cream into the house. I like to think we take a moderate, not an unhealthful, approach to eating."

A s long as you don't become junk-food vegetarians, snacking on sugary and fatty foods on occasion won't harm you. In fact, an argument could be made that a very rigid vegetarian diet is unhealthful, while a looser vegetarian diet overflows with goodness for body, mind and soul. Some rigid vegetarian diets, such as an extreme Zen macrobiotic diet, may lack vital nutrients; others might be harmful psychologically because the adherents work toward their idea of "perfection." And no diet is perfect.

As you make your food choices, remember that you're a very persuasive example to your children. Some research has revealed that vegetarianism is caught, not taught. Vegetarians influence their children and other people in their lives to eat better by the examples they set. In one study, 63 percent of nearly six hundred respondents to a survey said they stopped eating meat because of exposure to a vegetarian.

Knowing this, ask yourself whether you want your children to follow in your footsteps toward the snack cabinet. If yes, fine. If not, make dietary changes soon. Your example nearly dictates how your children will eat in the decades to come.

Healthful Fast Food

Whether your family's traveling the interstate on vacation or wants some quick vegetarian food, fast-food restaurants beckon. For every McDonald's, there's a Burger King or Wendy's within a few hundred yards. Like it or not, fast-food restaurants are a fact of life. Here are some healthful options.

Burger King: Order a vegetarian Whopper, light on (or without) mayonnaise. Most franchises have a key on their cash registers for this request, even though it's not mentioned on the menu. Other picks: garden salad, side salad and baked potato.

Hardee's: Other than salads and pancakes, there are few healthful choices available.

McDonald's: Healthful options are thin here too. The best bets: hotcakes, salads, yogurt and fat-free muffins where available.

Roy Rogers: The only slightly substantial healthful choices are pancakes, salads and yogurt.

Taco Bell: Go for a bean burrito, minus sour cream.

Wendy's: Possibly the best choice, this franchise offers fairly complete do-it-yourself salad bars in which you may make your own burritos with tortillas, refried beans and Spanish rice, top pasta with tomato sauce or load up on lettuce and other vegetables. Other options: prepackaged salads and baked potatoes.

Note: Top your salads, pancakes and potatoes wisely, avoiding excessive fat and sugar.

TV SEDUCTION

"My preteens watch their fair share of television, including sitcoms in which the stars eat junky snacks and commercials that make sugary cereals sound like health food. How influential is TV on kids' eating habits?

Very influential. So says the Center for Science in the Public Interest (CSPI), a consumer advocacy group based in Washington, D.C. The average child sees 350,000 to 400,000 television commercials by the time he or she graduates from high school. Assaulted by commercials and hoodwinked by television sitcoms as well as movies, children pick up a skewed view of what society thinks is best to eat.

A study conducted in 1994 gives reason for health-minded parents to shiver. After watching 104 hours of prime-time and Saturday morning TV and scoring all food-related incidents on the shows, not including commercials, it was found that junky food took the cake. Fat-rich foods, sweets and fat-rich protein foods were depicted in these percentages: 21.3, 14.7 and 13.0 respectively. Vegetables accounted for only 8.8 percent of the food-related incidents, and fruits managed a mere 3.5 percent.

Now let's add in the commercials. A pre-Christmas survey by CSPI in 1992 found that food commercials accounted for 29 percent of the 362 commercials. Of these commercials, nearly half (49 percent) pushed breakfast cereal, and the remainder delighted their young audience with promises of fast food, candy, drinks/chocolate syrup, milk and cookies. The single public service announcement among the commercials promoted fresh vegetables but did not discourage kids from eating fat- and sugar-laden foods.

Equally troublesome is the consequence-free slant of the programming. The characters in TV shows and commercials may down sodas and chomp on chips, but very few are overweight. The message is clear: Enjoy these exciting foods and live well. But it ain't the truth.

Parents can help uncover the lies by watching television with their children and educating them about the sneaky tactics advertisers use to lure their young viewers. Most children under five cannot differentiate between commercials and programs. Slightly older kids can learn that advertisers and programmers are playing mind games with them. You could also place a limit on television viewing.

TEASING FROM A PARENT

"My husband pokes fun at my daughter and me for eating meatless meals. He doesn't mean harm but his comments upset my daughter."

T easing can hurt a child deeply. How deeply depends in part on the sensitivity of your daughter and her overall relationship with her father. Since she has communicated her displeasure at your husband's bumbling attempts at humor, it would be best for him to lay off the comments.

Living in a home where one parent is a vegetarian and the other is not has its challenges. Some parents are able to use their differences in eating habits constructively by showing respect toward each other and communicating the value of differences. But when one parent— whether the meat eater or the vegetarian—harasses the other, even if the harassment is mild and seemingly good-natured, some children feel in the middle. It's possible your husband is using humor to cover up fear. He may feel rejection because you and your daughter are vegetarian. Ask him. You might find that he needs reassurance that you aren't pulling away from him. Hopefully, out of love for your daughter, your husband will choose his words more carefully, especially at this time, when most preteens are struggling with numerous changes.

BECOMING A VEGAN

"We've followed a near-vegetarian diet for years. My daughter now says she wants to be a vegan. Doesn't she need eggs and dairy products during adolescence?"

A vegan goes a few steps further with her vegetarian diet, omitting eggs and dairy products. Is it nutritious? Yes, it can be. Vegans get ample protein and other nutrients, except for vitamin B_{12} unless fortified foods are eaten.

Your daughter doesn't need eggs or dairy products. She can get her protein and calcium from plant foods. Of course, a diet pumped up with sugar, fat and junk food is unhealthful, just as it would be for a meat eater.

Encourage her to eat a varied diet and to take in enough calories—which shouldn't be a problem if she's listening to her hunger signals—and she'll be just fine. Also ask her why she has decided to be a vegan. Most vegans cite animal rights as their number-one reason for choosing to skip all animal products. As long as you don't sound like you're interrogating your daughter, she will probably open up and you'll have a chance to get to know her better as she heads into adolescence.

Later, if your daughter changes her mind and has a hankering for cheese pizza, so be it. She might find that she wavers between a vegetarian and a vegan diet, as some vegetarians do. Either way, she's set on a road toward lifelong health.

Still Struggling with Relatives

"I'm at my wit's end. My two preteen girls have been mostly vegetarian after I cleaned up our diet several years ago, but it seems that my parents haven't gotten the message. When we eat at their house, they usually serve a meat dish with a buttery vegetable side dish along with some white bread. The girls end up eating what they're served because they're hungry. I can't blame them. But I'm disappointed in my parents."

Unsupportive family members can make life miserable for new and longtime vegetarians. Only 10 percent of vegetarians responding to a survey about family relationships reported that their family members were supportive. Most family members are opposed to the change in eating habits or are indifferent. So take heart that you are not alone.

Now that your children are older, they can make their wishes known. You don't have to speak for them. However, they'll watch you carefully as you navigate through these waters of dietary differences with their grandparents. You're their role model. No matter your decision in handling this impasse with your folks—talking to them about healthful food choices, giving them recipes, bringing a dish to share, having them over for dinner at your house, where you dictate the menu—be sure to clearly communicate to your daughters how proud you are that they're making healthful choices for themselves. Your comforting words will be dearest to their hearts.

7

On Their Own— Almost

"**W**ho am I?" That's the question foremost on your teen's mind. While navigating her teen years, she needs to separate from you emotionally, but she will hold on to many of the core values she's learned since childhood. Even if your daughter ate meat on occasion in her grade school or preteen years, she could very well return to her vegetarian beginnings in her teens.

Some teens like the idea of being vegetarian because it sets them apart from the crowd. It may be a form of rebellion—a healthful form, but rebellion just the same. Even kids who've never dabbled in meatless meals may announce to their folks that they're vegetarian. Usually their parents are suspicious and unsupportive at first.

But research shows that the majority of teens believe the vegetarian diet is "in." Though most teens lack family support to become vegetarian, your daughter has you on her side. She might make decisions you don't agree with and demand her freedom, but she still hungers for your unconditional love. She needs you, now more than ever.

JOINING THE VEG CROWD

"When I attended high school, no one I knew was vegetarian. My daughter has several friends who don't eat meat. Is vegetarianism a new trend among teens?"

Yep. The kids of the Thirteenth Generation—so dubbed by Ian Howe, author of *13th Gen: Abort, Retry, Ignore, Fail?*—are showing deep concern for the world. Though some teens hold tight to apathy, trend watchers have noticed several positive trends: Many teens share environmental concerns, they search for spiritual answers for the meaning of life and they are repulsed by abuse toward animals.

Here are some stats. According to Teenage Research Unlimited, Northbrook, Illinois, more than 80 percent of teens say it's "in" to care about the environment. A group named YES! (Youth for Environmental Sanity) brings its message to about three hundred high schools in some twenty-five states each year. This troupe of young activists performs a game-show-style skit, presents a slide show on issues ranging from topsoil erosion to dangerous holes in the ozone and lauds the vegetarian diet.

The New York–based BrainReserve has noted that teens are getting more spiritual. To them, the world seems so messed up that only God can turn things right side up. Teens' ethical concerns are sometimes expressed through compassion for animals. Though no one has kept count of the numbers, animal rights groups for teens have been popping up all over the country. A magazine for concerned teens, *How on Earth!* gives the grizzly details about the conditions under which many factory farm animals live.

Most telling is a poll by teenage Research Unlimited: More than one in four teens describe being vegetarian as "in." No hard data exist to show how many teens are vegetarian. The data simply have not been gathered. The most comprehensive survey on vegetarians—specifically adult vegetarians—showed that 6.7 percent of adult Americans describe themselves as vegetarian. Every indication points to an even higher percentage for teens.

Here's a telltale sign: Though adult vegetarians cite health as their top reason for being vegetarian, teens in general say concern for the planet draws them to a meatless diet. The significance? Reasons other than health—environmental concerns, compassion for animals and spirituality—have staying power. People who are vegetarians for reasons beyond health tend to stick with their meatless choice.

Some veg teens have been accused of going through a phase, but trend watchers say this movement toward the vegetarian diet shows no signs of stopping.

"Six months ago, my seventeen-year-old son got involved with an animal rights group for teens and stopped eating meat. I thought his vegetarian diet was just a passing thing, but he's serious."

When actress Sara Gilbert, who not only plays a vegetarian on the TV sitcom *Roseanne* but also is one in real life, wore a T-shirt emblazoned with the words "Meat Stinks," she spoke for her generation. Today's teen vegetarians are sick of the status quo and they want change.

Teens still think they're invincible, so health arguments don't persuade them to cut back on meat and junk food. Rather, stories of what truly happens in factory farms and how meat eating ravages the planet cause them to think twice about inhaling a sausage pizza. Though the vast majority of teens eat Big Macs without regret, some of their chums are going green.

And these young vegetarians are serious. Some even take their message beyond their homes and their circle of friends and trumpet the pros of being vegetarian to a larger population. Witness the growing number of vegetarian groups and animal rights groups for teens. Other young vegetarians rally their schools to offer vegetarian alternatives at lunch—and some have succeeded.

As a parent of a veg teen, you might think your son is rebelling against you and you alone. But that's not likely the case. His involvement in an animal rights group suggests that his eyes have been opened to what he believes is a more compassionate lifestyle. When kids break out the tofu burgers, it's natural for parents to wonder what gives. But try not to see your son's vegetarian diet as a rejection of family values.

In his own way, he's showing concern for the world. And who can argue against that?

UNCONCERNED ABOUT HEALTH

"I'm proud that my teenage son is continuing his vegetarian beginnings, but he couldn't care less about his health. He inhales a bag of chips and a Coke every day, and says, 'Don't worry, Mom.' "

You're not alone. Vegetarian kids who ate healthful diets through their grade school years under the watchful eyes of their parents often junk out on junk food in their teens. Blood cholesterol levels, high blood pressure or excess sodium means next to nothing to teens. Some teens might worry about their weight because they're concerned about their appearance. But that's about as far as their health concerns go.

Remember the adage that you can lead a horse to water but you can't force it to drink? So it is with soon-to-be adults. You can offer whole-grain breakfast cereals, fruits for snacking and good meals (translate: delicious *and* nutritious). You can ban junk food from your home. You can encourage your teen's healthful eating habits, but you can't *control* them.

If his idea of a good lunch is a combo of chips, cookies, fries and Coke, your words of dietary wisdom may fall on deaf ears. He just isn't interested in health. Even many teens who are into sports eat their fair share of junk food. With a hero like Michael Jordan stuffing McDonald's burgers in his face on TV commercials, the lesson from M. J. is do what you want—no consequences.

That's hardly the truth. But, fortunately, there's reassuring news: The diets of vegetarian teens more closely conform to the government's recommendations to increase intakes of complex carbohydrates, vegetables and fruits than do the diets of their meat-eating friends. They also eat less junk food.

So though you may feel discouraged, don't throw in the dish towel. Continue to offer good foods, knowing that your example will eventually stick in his mind. You do make a difference.

GOING TOO FAR?

"Our teen not only has become a vegan but also has stopped wearing leather and using body-care products with animal ingredients. Is she becoming too extreme?"

Some people think veganism is extreme; others believe that the diet and lifestyle are just right. But because vegans are a drop in the bucket compared to the number of total U.S. vegetarians (with 4 percent of adult vegetarians describing themselves as vegan), they are often met with skepticism, doubt and a barrage of questions—even from fellow vegetarians.

The simple definition of vegan is a person who consumes no animal flesh, eggs or dairy products. Yet the ethics and philosophy of the diet go far beyond diet. Besides not eating foods of animal origin, vegans in general do not wear or use anything that comes from an animal, including leather, fur, silk, feathers, wool, cosmetics, body-care products, medications and fertilizers that include bonemeal, dried blood and other slaughterhouse by-products. Thankfully, for people who come in close range of teens, many supermarkets and natural food stores sell shampoos, deodorants and other pleasant-smelling toiletries that contain no animal products and have not been tested on animals.

Vegans choose a way of living that avoids exploitation and embraces life to the full. Even philosopher and theologian Albert Schweitzer watched his every move, literally. He avoided stepping on a single ant, lest he take its life.

But—surprise, surprise—it's all but impossible to be a vegan. Even if your daughter reads every product label, deciphering each chemical name to determine whether the ingredient is of animal origin, she can't eliminate animal products from her world. The only way for her to make a break from animal products is to build a special home and furnish it with materials she acquires from nature, grow and make her own food and depend on no transportation except for her own two feet.

That's because animal by-products are in the steel of cars, rubber-soled shoes, videos, varnish, carpentry glue, bricks, home insulation and house paint, plus many, many other things you wouldn't think have a connection to animals. The point is, your teen can't be a vegan in the strictest sense, try as she might.

So the question to ask yourself: Is your daughter so consumed by her vegan choice that she's making life horrible for herself and your family? If not, let her be. If so, then choose to either ride out her intense interest in veganism or discuss with her ways to ease up her demands on herself and the people nearest her.

Though veganism might be considered extreme by the world at large, the diet can be healthful, environmentally sound and compassionate. Science says so.

CRAZY ABOUT ANIMALS?

"Our two teens are very active in a local youth animal rights group. I've heard so many negative news stories about animal rights activists that I'm concerned they might be encouraged to break into research labs to free animals or do something equally crazy."

The animal rights movement has suffered a public-relations night-mare. A handful of activists have bombed research labs and trashed the offices of scientists, but most animal rights group members steer clear of violence and lawlessness. As with any cause, there are some extremists who may give a bad name to the movement as a whole.

The only way to know what your teens are doing is to ask them. In a nonthreatening manner, engage them in a conversation about their animal rights group. Try questions like, "What do your animal rights friends like to do when you get together?" or "How does the animal rights group plan to help animals?" If you suspect wrongdoing, a direct approach may be best. "Have you done anything dangerous?" is one possible query.

The chances are great that your teens' animal rights group is effecting change through peaceful methods: educating others via newsletters, taking part in letter-writing campaigns and supporting boycotts of body-care items containing animal by-products. In the unlikely case that your teens are involved in a group whose methods are questionable, encourage them to join a different group that truly reflects the peaceful spirit of being vegetarian.

DATING

"My son's going to a movie and dinner with a new girlfriend. She doesn't know he's a vegetarian and he fears she'll dump him if she finds out. What's the best way for him to break the news?"

To tell or not to tell? That's the question on the minds of many vegetarians—whether in their teens or in later life—when they start dating a new person. A teen especially has a need to be understood and to belong, so he might fear how others will interpret his lifestyle. He may wonder, "Will my date make fun of my vegetarian diet or will she confess that she detests meat too?"

When beginning a dating relationship, it's not necessary to "break the news" right away. Your son and his friend can select an eating place that has many vegetarian selections. Italian and Asian restaurants are always good bets. He can order his food without giving an explanation for his choice of entrée.

Still, if he plans to continue the relationship, he will probably want to tell her about his values, hoping she shares similar ones. If not a vegetarian diet, then she might feel as passionate about saving the planet as he does. Eventually, he'll want to know if she'll accept him and his vegetarian diet.

That said, the best way to break the news is to bring up the subject in the course of conversation. He might say, "I've never liked meat," "Let's go to such and such a restaurant. It's got great vegetarian food," or "Have you ever met a vegetarian?" From these remarks, his new girlfriend will probably guess his dietary preference. With so many teens considering the vegetarian diet to be "in," she might think he's ultra-cool.

And, as you know and as he'll learn, if she dumps him simply because he's a vegetarian, his new girlfriend was never a true friend anyway. So what may seem a loss at the time is actually a door opening to new possible friendships with people who value your son as he is.

CLEARING UP ACNE

"My fifteen-year-old son has been a vegetarian for several years and now is battling a case of acne. What foods can he add or remove from his diet to clear his skin?"

T he link between diet and acne is murky, with some health practitioners believing fatty and allergenic foods may worsen this no-fun condition and others insisting that diet has nothing to do with acne. Before considering a few tips for your son, an accurate description of this condition is in order.

Acne—pimples or zits—on the face, neck and back occurs when the hair follicles in the skin become plugged with dead skin and oil secreted by sebaceous glands. This results in blackheads if the pore remains open (the "black" isn't dirt; it's caused by oxidation of the oil) or whiteheads if the pore is blocked. Sometimes a cyst forms under the skin and becomes red when infected.

About three out of four teens have some acne. Acne is most prevalent in adolescents due to hormonal changes that stimulate their sebaceous glands. Acne is related to heredity. But it may have other causes.

Diet: Though there's little hard data proving that consuming chocolate, cola, pizza or greasy food causes or aggravates acne, a *low-fat* vegetarian diet remains your son's first weapon in battling acne. Excess fat contributes to an increase of hormones in the body and can affect the secretions of the sebaceous glands. A healthful vegetarian diet also helps fight infection, and pimples are infections.

A minority of teens discover that certain foods, such as those named above, do indeed worsen their acne. To find out if certain foods are wreaking havoc with your son's skin, eliminate them from his diet for a week or two and observe whether his complexion improves. If his condition lessens, great. Keep the aggravating foods out of his diet. Or test specific foods by adding one at a time, noting whether his skin seems affected.

Some physicians believe that supplements of zinc and vitamins E and A may help skin troubles. If you choose to go the supplement route, be sure your son doesn't overdo them; taking too much can cause nutritional imbalances and may be toxic in high amounts.

Beyond food: Stress can contribute to skin troubles. Picking at skin may aggravate the condition. So can the use of oily lotions or oil-based cosmetics spread on the affected areas. It's best to use water-based skin-care products. Sunshine and physical activities help.

Because acne can cause scarring, both physical and psychological, teens who have more serious conditions may benefit by turning to a skin-care specialist. Doctors can prescribe medications, such as a vitamin A derivative, to improve complexions.

Fortunately, nature is on your son's side. As he ages and his sebaceous glands become less active, his skin will clear up. Time may be his best medicine.

HEALTHFUL WEIGHT LOSS

"Our seventeen-year-old daughter told us that she's become a vegetarian because she wants to lose weight. She's a little overweight, but I wonder whether she should be on a diet at all."

Dieting to lose weight makes sense for a teen who's overweight, especially in light of two truths: First, an overweight teen can suffer a poor self-image and feelings of worthlessness that may affect her for years, and, second, she may be setting herself up for a life of battling the bulge if she's carrying or gaining excess weight as she enters adulthood.

A vegetarian weight-loss plan is ideal for losing excess pounds and keeping them off. Vegetarian foods tend to be rich in fiber and low in fat. When your daughter makes low-fat selections, she can eat enough food to fill her up, snuffing any desire to scarf down high-calorie snacks. What's more, a gram of fat has nine hefty calories, compared to the four calories in a gram of either carbohydrate or protein. Dietary fat is not only more than twice as calorie-dense as carbohydrate and protein but is also more fattening. Several studies have shown that fat calories slip easily into fat stores, while carbohydrate and protein calories do not.

Though fat is most fattening, the equation for weight loss remains true: To lose body fat, burn more calories than you eat. (See "Why Huff and Puff?" page 126.) Discourage your daughter from trying crash diets or skipping meals, which may set off a starve-and-binge cycle that's bad news. Rather, encourage her to eat breakfast, lunch and dinner as well as a snack or two each day. Splurging on a favorite treat occasionally is fine. The point isn't deprivation; it's learning life-long healthful eating habits.

To get off to a good start, your daughter may need to familiarize herself with the fat contents of her usual foods so she can make healthful adjustments in her diet. (See "The Fat-Gram Counter," page 215.) A respectable weekly weight loss is one or two pounds a week. Quicker weight loss may mean she's not eating enough food to get adequate nutrients. Moreover, weight loss at a steady but sure pace is longer lasting, studies show.

Almost anyone can shed pounds, but *maintaining* proper weight matters most. Translate: Eat low-fat meals that are satisfying and allow an occasional treat. Then your daughter will have motivation to eat right.

"Our teen has had trouble with eating disorders. She had been eating right this past year, but now she's become a vegetarian. I'm wondering whether her new diet is a mask for another eating disorder."

The sad truth is a number of young people with eating disorders hide behind the vegetarian diet to mask their problems with food. Though following a healthful vegetarian diet is an excellent way to maintain proper weight and avoid heart disease, cancer and many other deadly illnesses down the line, the diet can be used to rationalize rigid food choices.

For instance, a teenage girl may describe herself as a vegetarian, making it appear that she's doing something good for herself when in fact she's passing up not only the meat but also the vegetarian foods she needs for her health. When asked why she didn't eat the mashed potatoes served at dinner, she might respond, "Oh, I couldn't. It has too much butter in it." Her answer sounds reasonable, but it may be deceptive. She may have skipped potatoes because she didn't want to eat, period.

In the past decade, the number of eating disorder cases has increased about 50 percent. Some people suffer from *anorexia nervosa* (in which they eat so little that they face near starvation); others have *bulimia nervosa* (in which they binge and purge by vomiting and using laxatives). There are other forms of eating disorders, such as chronic overeating.

To help you spot an eating disorder, ask your daughter why she is a vegetarian. If her reason is to lose or maintain her weight, your concern is warranted. Also note whether she eats a variety of foods (good) or just a few (not good). If she's restrictive in her eating and shows other signs of rigidity, such as exercising compulsively, it's possible she's fallen back into her old, destructive ways. Seriously consider seeking outside help.

With eating disorders becoming more common, even among girls as young as ten or eleven years old, parents are smart to keep an eye on their children's diet, vegetarian or not.

VEG DORMS

"My vegetarian teen is making plans for college. How do we locate a college that serves vegetarian food?"

With an increasing number of colleges and universities offering vegetarian options in dormitory cafeterias, your teen should have little trouble finding food. At the University of California–Berkeley, for instance, the food service has dished up vegetarian food for about eight years and recently added vegan (no animal products whatsoever) to its offerings. Still, your son will need to do a fair amount of research because some institutions of higher learning still serve hamburger surprise instead of healthful foods.

To locate a college that caters to vegetarians, he can start with his list of the colleges he'd most like to attend. Then encourage him to start dialing. He can get the phone number of the college ombudsman or the food service and ask whether the dorm cafeterias serve a vegetarian meal at each meal. He should ask specific questions to avoid confusion. One possible confusion is the word *vegetarian*. Some people think vegetarians eat poultry and fish.

If he learns that the dorms do serve vegetarian meals, he ought to follow up with questions regarding the types of meals. Are the veg meals hot entrées, or is the extent of the dorm's meatless offerings some bagels at breakfast and a salad bar at lunch and dinner? He also needs to ask whether the hot vegetarian entrées ever include chicken or beef broth, or other "hidden" meats.

Some colleges have separate vegetarian cafeterias, where only meatless meals are served. He can ask how he can get a spot in a dorm with a vegetarian cafeteria. But he still needs to ask the follow-up questions.

You and your son will find that he can locate a college that serves vegetarian food, but asking specific questions and getting detailed answers is paramount *before* you send in the application with the check. College is an investment in many ways—time and finances, to name two. So insist on knowing the food situation in the dorms up front.

Why Huff and Puff?

Sitting at desks all day, flopping in front of the TV, talking on the phone for hours. These typical teen activities burn minimal calories and don't strengthen the body. Yet young people—and their parents—need exercise for overall health. Diet is one important aspect, exercise is another.

Fitness researchers now push a balanced workout of aerobics *and* strength training. They are the flip sides of the same fitness coin. Aerobic exercise is any steady-state activity like cycling, swimming or walking. It works the heart, improving cardiovascular health. Except for swimming and rowing, aerobic exercise does little to strengthen the upper body. Strength training encompasses many types of exercise—from calisthenics and weight lifting to working out with weight machines and oversize rubber bands—all of which work various muscle groups.

Getting strong is easier than you might think. In fact, two twenty-minute strength-training sessions a week are all you need. Each session should consist of eight to ten exercises (one set per exercise, eight to twelve repetitions per set) to condition the major muscle groups (shoulders, chest, back, arms, legs and abdomen).

Though the obvious result of strength training is stronger muscles, the reasons to curl biceps go far beyond a quest for sheer power. Indeed, fitness experts say avoiding regular strength-training exercises—especially those for the upper body, where 65 percent of the body's muscles are located—almost guarantees a flabby, injury-prone, decrepit future.

Here's a rundown of the main muscle-up benefits.

Burn, Baby, Burn

Muscles are the key to a revved-up metabolism, the pace at which the body burns calories. The more muscle you have, the more calories you burn, even when watching television. How so? Even when you're at rest, your muscles are very active on a biochemical level, guzzling calories twenty-four hours a day. Pound for pound, muscle burns about fifty more calories a day than fat. So adding just two pounds of muscle will consume an extra one hundred calories a day. You don't get this same effect from aerobic exercise.

On the Inside

Muscling up also means stronger ligaments and tendons and denser bones. Stronger ligaments and tendons mean a reduced risk of sustaining injuries and accidents because you have better balance and can react more quickly. Strength training increases bone density by placing beneficial stress on bones. This is helpful during the teen years and beyond: People with denser bones are less likely to suffer osteoporosis, a bone-thinning disease.

Heart Smarts

Fitness experts are mixed when it comes to whether strength training has cardiovascular benefits. Some give a qualified yes, others say definitely no. But they agree on one point: To become aerobically fit, aerobic exercise is the top pick; for strong muscles, strength-train.

At Oregon Health Sciences University in Portland, researchers have measured indicators, such as blood cholesterol levels, that suggest improved cardiovascular function in people who strength-train regularly. In one study, competitive bodybuilders showed a rise in high-density lipoprotein, or "good" cholesterol, and a drop in low-density lipoprotein, or "bad" cholesterol.

Super Self-Esteem

Though the psychological benefits of strength training aren't as well researched as those of aerobics, surveys have shown that a boost in self-image and confidence goes hand in hand with getting stronger. Fitness experts agree: Strength training boosts self-esteem.

And what teen couldn't use a dose of that?

CHOOSING WORDS WISELY

"I'm glad my teens are vegetarians. In their own way, they're showing respect for life. Unfortunately, their rhetoric can get quite hurtful. I wish they'd be more gentle in their speaking when trying to win converts to their vegetarian way."

Speak the truth with love. This motto makes sense in all dealings of life, though it can be difficult to be loving toward people who are different or when one feels passionate about a cause.

Confrontation rarely achieves the desired ends of the confronter who wants to win converts. Harsh words usually fall on deaf ears or can backfire, prompting meat eaters to defend themselves. A better way is being an example of healthful living and remaining open to answer questions about the vegetarian diet. Encourage your kids to try this approach. They'll find it works.

Interestingly, most vegetarians do not want to confront people who don't share their dietary choice. According to a 1992 survey, only one out of ten vegetarians is bothered so much by meat eating that they'd confront a steak lover. The majority (66 percent) say they are not bothered by meat eating. The remainder are bothered but wouldn't confront.

In fact, vegetarians are far more likely to confront someone doing harm to the environment, with 69 percent of the survey respondents reporting they would speak up. The findings of the survey suggest that vegetarians in general take an accepting view toward nonvegetarians.

Vegetarians are also seen as helpful. According to the survey, 63 percent of vegetarians said that someone had asked them for advice on nutrition, food or health in the previous six months simply because they were vegetarian.

The take-home message: By speaking the truth in love, vegetarian teens can make a difference. So can you.

8

A Broader Perspective: Why Be a Vegetarian?

S urveys indicate that twenty thousand Americans become vegetarians *each week*. The hope of improved health draws most new
adult vegetarians. Though there is no comprehensive study of why
kids go green, informal surveys suggest that they give little thought
to health. Let's be serious: If you were eleven years old, would you
junk the junk and eat healthful foods for fear you might get cancer
or heart disease by the time you're a senior citizen?

Kids embrace other reasons to be vegetarian, including concern
for the planet, animals and starving people. Some kids are vegetarian
out of spiritual convictions.

Interestingly, health-minded adult vegetarians often come to
adopt these other reasons supporting their vegetarian choice. Call it
the domino effect. As new and aspiring vegetarians learn more about
the effect of their food choices, they want to know more. And the
more they know, the more reasons they discover in favor of the vegetarian diet.

Here are the main reasons kids "veg out."

ENVIRONMENTAL CONCERNS

Some vegetarians choose a meatless diet because they consider it kinder to the planet. Here's a collection of statistics from a variety of sources that back up their beliefs. The numbers might startle you.

Gallons of water needed to produce 1 pound of beef: 2,500
Gallons of water needed to produce 1 pound of wheat: 25
Percent of U.S. water used in some phase of livestock production: 50
Average amount of water required daily by an average meat-eater:
    4,200 gallons. By an ovo-lacto vegetarian: 1,200 gallons. By a vegan: 300 gallons.
Amount of U.S. topsoil lost to date: about ⅔
U.S. topsoil loss linked to livestock raising: 85 percent
Amount of waste produced every second by animals raised for human consumption: 125 tons
Water pollution linked to waste from livestock, including manure, pesticides and fertilizers: more than 50 percent
Tropical rain forest deforestation linked to livestock raising: more than 50 percent
Rate of species extinction caused by tropical rain forest destruction: about 1,000 per year
Amount of forest lost for every hamburger produced from livestock that graze on land that was Central American forest: 55 square feet
U.S. grain fed to cattle and other livestock: more than 70 percent
Americans who consider themselves environmentalists: about 75 percent
Average amount of meat eaten by an average American each year: 114 pounds. By a vegetarian: 0

If these facts astound you, consider this: Modern animal raising is designed to be efficient, to get more output from less input. The inputs—clean air and water, government grazing land, energy and feed grains—are either free or cheap. The negative outputs, such as topsoil loss and air and water pollution, cost very little to the producers. They lack strong incentives to clean up their messes.

And the trend is continuing. Says Joan Dye Gussow, professor of

How Kids Can Save the Planet

1. Eat vegetarian, of course. Every time your child chooses a veggie burger over a hamburger, she conserves topsoil, keeps the air and water cleaner and rescues a portion of rain forest.
2. Recycle. Participating in your community's recycling program, which usually includes paper, cardboard, aluminum, glass and plastic, shows your child that you want to avoid the unnecessary production of new products whenever possible. Assign him a portion of the recycling tasks, such as hauling the recyclables to the curb for pickup. Here's an amazing fact: 84 percent of a typical household's waste, including food scraps, yard waste, paper and cans, can be recycled.
3. Turn off the water. When your child washes his hands or brushes his teeth, encourage him to use as little water as possible. Believe it or not, allowing the water to run while brushing teeth wastes up to five gallons. If you figure two brushings a day, one child can waste about 3,650 gallons of water a year.
4. Bike instead of ride. Weather permitting, ride bikes with your kids when you head to the park, the post office or another local destination. Driving wastes energy and pollutes the air. And biking is more fun.
5. Donate toys to a worthy cause. When your child gets tired of a toy, give it to the Salvation Army or another nonprofit organization that will recycle it. Toys thrown in the garbage usually end up at a landfill.
6. Hold onto balloons. Helium balloons released into the air can harm and even kill animals and fish, which might mistake them for food or ingest by accident.
7. Pick up litter. Talk to your kids about the reasons littering is bad. Encourage them to keep wrappers and other garbage until they locate a trash can.
8. Join a youth environmental group. If your child doesn't know of one, contact your local vegetarian society, which should have some leads.

nutrition education at Columbia University Teachers College in New York City and author of *Chicken Little, Tomato Sauce and Agriculture:* "It is clear that the rising appetite for meat around the world cannot be met without accelerating environmental damage." She has called for a sustainable diet. By "sustainable," she means a diet of foods that are organic and locally grown, and that are conscientiously chosen with the world in mind. She says that it's not enough to be concerned with personal health.

This planetary approach fits the mind-set of environmentally minded vegetarians. Yet it's been argued that the most ecological diet might require an integrated system that produces both animals and plants for human consumption because eliminating animals would decrease sustainability. If all this sounds confusing, know one sure fact: Your family's commitment to a vegetarian diet is environmentally sound today.

Maybe in a hundred or so years, when your descendants inhabit this earth and humans have recognized the destructiveness of animal agriculture, the story might be different. A sustainable diet that includes minimal amounts of meat might prove best for the planet. But, until then, you can't go wrong dining on delightful vegetarian cuisine.

Recommended reading for adults and older children:
Lappé, Frances Moore. *Diet for a Small Planet: 10th Anniversary Edition.* New York: Ballantine Books, 1986.
Rifkin, Jeremy. *Beyond Beef: The Rise and Fall of the Cattle Culture.* New York: Dutton, 1992.
Robbins, John. *Diet for a New America.* Walpole, N. H.: Stillpoint, 1987.

A great book for young readers:
Elkington, John, et al. *Going Green: A Kid's Handbook to Saving the Planet.* New York: Viking, 1990.

Plastic Toys and the Earth

When purchasing toys for your child, consider the environment. Most toys are made out of plastic, which takes hundreds of years to degrade, so discarded plastic toys usually end up in waste dumps. The manufacturing of plastic also releases volatile chemicals into the air, polluting the skies. Incinerating plastic also pollutes.

An alternative: Buy wooden or cloth toys.

If you desire, you could take your environmental concerns a step further: Plant trees—or donate money to a tree-planting charity—to replace the ones that are cut to make wooden toys.

COMPASSION FOR ANIMALS

You don't need to witness a slaughter to have compassion for animals. Vegetarians who embrace animal welfare or animal rights—terms that are often used interchangeably—have rarely seen the inside of a slaughterhouse or an animal factory farm. But like other Americans who hate to see a lion penned or an eagle caged, some vegetarians are sensitive to animal abuse, whether that abuse occurs at a slaughterhouse, a pet store, a zoo, a circus, a rodeo or wherever.

These vegetarians try to make a real difference, one forkful at a time, by choosing a meatless diet.

Animal factories aren't Old MacDonald's farms. They are economic ventures, where profit rules. The Humane Society of the United States, considered moderate in its views on animal welfare, objects to the systems of modern factory farming, which are abusive to animals. Many animals in factory farms are kept in overcrowded, unsanitary conditions (no wonder so many chickens carry salmonella!), fed drugs routinely and endure painful procedures, such as debeaking (in which the tip of chickens' beaks are sliced off with a knife, to keep them from cannibalizing each other). The sickening details go on.

Shortly after birth, most baby calves are taken from their mothers and are confined in individual crates so small that they cannot turn around. They are fed an iron-poor diet that makes them anemic and weak, so their flesh stays white, the preferred color of veal gourmands. The calves are slaughtered at about sixteen weeks of age and turn up on plates at restaurants and in packages in supermarkets. Because the dairy and veal industries are linked, some vegetarians choose not to consume dairy products.

Many pigs are kept in confinement systems too. The sows have the hardest life. Only a few weeks after piglets are born, they are taken away. Then the sows are artificially inseminated again and the cycle repeats.

Broiler chickens (the type people eat) call warehouses their home. Thousands of birds live in a single, windowless warehouse, where their total environment—lighting, feeding, space—is controlled. As the chicks grow and approach their market weight (about three and a half pounds), some die from stress and suffocation because there's little room to move, let alone flap their wings.

Laying hens may have the worst life. Three to five birds are crammed into each wire battery cage, measuring approximately ten

How Kids Can Make a Difference

❖ Join a youth animal rights group. These groups are becoming more prevalent. If you have trouble locating one, contact the nearest vegetarian society or natural food store. They might have information.

❖ Donate money to national animal rights groups. Your dollars make a difference in supporting programs that help animals.

❖ Visit and support places, such as wildlife centers and arboretums, that show respect toward animals. Avoid exploitive entertainment, such as rodeos and circuses.

❖ Read books about animals, particularly those in danger of extinction, to develop a better understanding of birds, reptiles, amphibians and mammals.

❖ Delight in a vegetarian diet. By choosing a meatless diet, you save the lives of animals.

inches by twelve inches by fourteen inches. The cages are stacked one on top of another. The hens do not have enough room to spread their wings or lay their eggs comfortably. They often try to cannibalize one another due to their high-stress environment. About 95 percent of eggs are produced by factory-farmed laying hens.

Relatively speaking, beef cattle bask in the glory of freedom—for a time. They spend part of their life on the range and the remainder in overcrowded feedlots, where they eat a concentrated diet to ready them for market.

Animal rights advocates contend that all animals raised for meat are exploited, even the few that are raised on family farms. But animal factories are only one part of the story. Animal rights advocates also have a bone to pick with medical research labs that use animals in laboratory experiments. Some of the experiments are hideous, causing animals pain and mutilation. Though the medical establishment supports experiments using animals for the benefits humans may receive, opponents say that animal experiments can produce faulty information because the physiologies of animals and humans differ substantially and because alternatives, such as computer models, are sometimes available.

Many animal rights advocates also have little good to say about rodeos, circuses, dog and horse racing and other enterprises that not only abuse animals but also pervert their natural behaviors. Dogs jumping through fiery hoops and chimps wearing clothes may seem funny and amazing. Yet these are distortions. They show no respect for the animals.

A change is in the works. People who've championed the cause of animal rights have seen victories. For instance, the use of animals in laboratory tests dropped 50 percent in the past decade, and many major cosmetic companies no longer test their products on animals. Despite the victories, infighting among animal rights advocates may threaten their cause. As with any movement, there are moderates and extremists who don't agree with each other's positions and tactics.

As individuals, however, vegetarians who choose a meatless diet out of compassion for animals *always* make a difference—even when the change comes one forkful at a time.

Recommended reading for adults and older children:

Mason, Jim. *Animal Factories Update*. New York: Crown, 1990.

Moran, Victoria. *Compassion: The Ultimate Ethic*. Great Britain: Thorsons Publishers, 1985.

Sharpe, Robert. *The Cruel Deception: The Use of Animals in Medical Research*. Great Britain: Thorsons Publishers, 1988.

Singer, Peter. *Animal Liberation: A New Ethics for Our Treatment of Animals*. New York: Avon Books, 1975.

GROUPS

These major national animal rights and welfare organizations, as well as other groups, have spearheaded programs, conducted campaigns and boycotted products in support of animals. Write to them for more information.

Farm Animal Reform Movement (FARM), Box 30654, Bethesda, MD 20824. Focus: Campaigning against animals used for food.

Farm Sanctuary, P.O. Box 150, Watkins Glen, NY 14891. Focus: Sheltering abused farm animals.

The Fund for Animals, 200 W. 57th St., New York, NY 10019. Focus: Supporting animals in general.

Humane Society of the United States, 2100 L St. NW, Washington, DC 20037. Focus: Protecting animals.

National Anti-Vivisection Society, 53 W. Jackson Blvd., Chicago, IL 60604. Focus: Campaigning against animal experimentation.

People for the Ethical Treatment of Animals (PETA), P.O. Box 42516, Washington, DC 20015. Focus: Supporting animals in general.

SAVING THE STARVING

TRUE OR FALSE:
By choosing a vegetarian diet, you help relieve world hunger.

The answer is true *and* false. Here's why. Though Western farming practices—especially the feeding of grain to cattle destined for slaughter—are wasteful, politics determines who gets food. Corrupt governments, for instance, have stolen relief donations of food meant for starving people and turned it into their profit. The root of world starvation isn't the lack of food availability, but politics and economics. In other words, the misuse of power. Scarcity is an illusion; our planet has the capacity to feed the world, *even if some people continue to eat meat*. So, in one respect, choosing a vegetarian diet cannot relieve world hunger.

However, some Third World people do go hungry because the steak "religion" has infiltrated their communities, forcing them to use their land for grazing and not for growing food. The cattle grazed on their land is slaughtered and exported to Western countries to satisfy the demands of the wealthy. Many Third World countries condone this practice, even though their people go hungry, in order to pay off huge debts. So if Westerners didn't want beef, which requires about sixteen pounds of grain to produce one pound of meat, then these Third World people could probably keep some of the grain for themselves and have enough to eat.

There's much more to the world hunger story. It doesn't stop at meat. American food companies have set up shop in foreign countries where they pay workers low wages for hard labor and figure they'll feed their families somehow.

The meat-centered diet may be incredibly wasteful. But even worse is the treatment of the dispossessed, the poor, the powerless, at the hands of the powerful. For more on this topic, read Frances Moore Lappé's and Joseph Collin's *Food First: Beyond the Myth of Scarcity* (Houghton Mifflin, 1977) and Frances Moore Lappé's *Diet for a Small Planet: 10th Anniversary Edition* (Ballantine Books, 1986).

THE SPIRITUAL SIDE

Seventh-Day Adventists, members of a Protestant denomination, pass up meat in adherence to a biblical principle that the body is a temple of the Holy Spirit and should be treated with reverence.

Jains, members of a Hindu sect, wear gauze masks when they leave their houses so they won't accidentally breathe in insects. Their religion mandates that they kill nothing, not even a bug.

Buddhists follow the teachings of Buddha, who lived several centuries before the birth of Christ, including his lessons on compassion for all life, and many choose a vegetarian path.

Eastern Orthodox monks living in Nebraska follow a vegan lifestyle out of love for God and his creation. They even put together a cookbook, *Simply Heavenly! The Monastery Vegetarian Cookbook.*

The list of people who choose a vegetarian diet for spiritual, sometimes called ethical, reasons goes on and on. They find support for their meatless choice in Scripture, ancient sacred text and religious tradition. Sometimes the support on which they rely is obscure; sometimes it's crystal-clear. Each of the five main religions—Christianity, Judaism, Hinduism, Buddhism and Islam—offers some basis for the vegetarian diet, usually growing out of compassion for all creation.

But some people who cite spiritual reasons say it just "feels right." They might rely on their own conscience and standards of right and wrong rather than depend on a particular religion's teachings. This gets deep and very personal, to be sure. Yet the question of right and wrong and its application to creation, including animals, is real to an unknown number of vegetarians. No study to date has specifically asked about spiritual reasons for being vegetarian. An imperfect indication is a 1992 survey in which 5 percent of American adults describing themselves as vegetarian cited "ethical reasons" as their single most important reason for becoming vegetarian. But because many vegetarians find spiritual reasons for their diet *after* they've chosen the meatless path, the numbers remain unclear.

What's certain is the strong commitment that "spiritual" vegetarians have to a meatless diet. Vegetarian Jews and Christians find heart in God's instruction to Adam and Eve in Genesis 1:29: "Then God said, 'I give you every seed-bearing plant on the face of the whole earth and every tree that has fruit with seed in it. They will be yours for food.' " This original dietary rule from God shows his intention for humans to be vegetarian, some vegetarian Jews and Christians believe.

A few scholars believe that Jesus himself was a vegetarian, citing ancient texts that suggest he was an Essene Jew; the Essenes supposedly did not slaughter living creatures. However, the Bible itself points to the contrary. It contains several references to Jesus eating fish (Luke 24:43) and catching or distributing fish. Jesus' main teaching was relationship—to love God, neighbor and self—and not diet. Though his peaceful words are in line with the compassionate philosophy of the vegetarian diet, there's no hard evidence he was vegetarian.

In the Eastern religious realm, some scholars of Islam say Muhammad was a vegetarian and recount the story when Muhammad awoke to find a cat sleeping on the sleeve of his robe and cut off the sleeve with a knife so the cat would not be disturbed from its slumber. However, there is no vegetarian tradition among Muslims.

Even Hindus have a history of eating meat with great delight. When there was a major upheaval in India in the sixth century B.C., leading to the formation of the Buddhist and Jain religions, Hinduism was deeply affected. The Hindus began to ascribe to the Buddhist belief of the sanctity of all life. Meat eating among Hindus took a downturn.

The world religions aside, spiritual reasons for a meatless diet interweave with other reasons, namely animal rights, environment and health. It's difficult to pull them apart because they are interconnected. Values such as compassion, good stewardship, balance, peace and justice touch every aspect of being vegetarian, whether one acknowledges it or not.

A wonderful word picture comes from Isaiah: "The wolf will live with the lamb, the leopard will lie down with the goat, the calf and the lion and the yearling together; and a little child will lead them" (11:6). Welcome to the peaceable kingdom.

Recommended reading for adults and older children:

Akers, Keith. *A Vegetarian Sourcebook: The Nutrition, Ecology and Ethics of a Natural Foods Diet.* Arlington, Va.: Vegetarian Press, 1983.

Linzey, Andrew. *Christianity and the Rights of Animals.* New York: Crossroads, 1987.

Linzey, Andrew, and Regan, Tom. *Animals and Christianity: A Book of Reading.* New York: Crossroads, 1988.

Moran, Victoria. *Compassion: The Ultimate Ethic.* Great Britain: Thorsons Publishers, 1985.

Rosen, Steven. *Food for the Spirit: Vegetarianism and the World Religions.* Poway, Calif.: Bala Books, 1987.

Schwartz, Richard. *Judaism and Vegetarianism.* Marblehead, Mass.: Micah Publications, 1988.

Now that you know the reasons why kids become vegetarian, you're in a better position to parent well. If your child has recently announced she's a vegetarian, you can better understand her vegetarian choice. If you're trying to convince your family to become vegetarian, you can appeal to their concerns for the planet and animals.

But it's not enough to know about the vegetarian choice. Equally important, you and your family need good food. That means absolutely wonderful meatless creations. In the next section, you'll learn about making satisfying meals and you'll be served up dozens of family-oriented recipes. Your kids will love them. So will you.

PART II

Meal Planning, Menus and Recipes

9

Making a Real Meal

Customized for your family, these recipes put the fun back into food. They're easy to prepare, and they play up nutrition. Equally important, these recipes emphasize good taste. No lentil-nut loaves. No rabbit food. No nutritional yeast or wheat germ sprinkled on *everything*. Even finicky kids and meat-eating spouses like these recipes. (I tested them on my kindergartner and my husband, chucking the ones that got a "yuck" and keeping the "yummy" ones.)

But recipes by themselves don't make a meal. You need a plan. Before I share ideas for planning menus, a word about making the transition into eating vegetarian.

You may have wondered: Should my family, whether it boasts three or eight members, become vegetarian overnight or gradually? Both approaches have their advantages and disadvantages. When family members commit to the vegetarian diet all of a sudden, they might experience improvements in health from the get-go and have greater incentive to stick with their meatless choice. (This is truer for grown-ups than children because adults are more likely to have health problems that respond to dietary changes.) However, saying good-bye to favorite meat foods can be hard; some family members may slip up and give up. In contrast, a gradual approach allows the family to get used to vegetarian dishes while feasting on meat occasionally. The disadvantage is that some family members may never make the switch to a totally meatless diet, preferring near-vegetarian status.

If your family is struggling with becoming vegetarian—or if you're already vegetarian but want to make further dietary improvements— I urge you to persevere. Your family not only will enjoy health benefits now and in the decades to come but also will embark on a culinary adventure. The average American diet is limited to meat, dairy products, a few vegetables and fruits and some bread, and is spiked with junk food. In a word, boring.

A healthful vegetarian diet? That's a tale worth telling.

THE MAKING OF A MEAL

"What do vegetarians eat?" This common question underscores a sad revelation: The Western concept of a meal as meat in the center of the plate, with a side dish or two and maybe dessert, is ingrained in our culture. When the meat disappears, many people feel lost.

The truth is that vegetarians eat *everything* but the meat. Everything means grains such as rice, bulgur, couscous, barley, wheat and amaranth; vegetables beyond green beans (think kohlrabi, jicama, artichokes, kale and collards); fruits of every imaginable color and flavor (honeydew, star fruit, kiwi, berries and citrus); and a hundred varieties of legumes (including the familiar chickpeas and lentils as well as rattlesnake beans and adzukis) and soy foods made from soybeans—plus dairy products and eggs if desired.

Most vegetarians discover an amazing quantity and quality of foods when they go green. It's not a matter of finding something to replace the meat, but opening oneself up to a new and inspiring way of cooking. Here are some menu-planning ideas.

❖ Choose vegetarian versions of your favorite meat-containing meals. Examples are spinach lasagna, vegetable stir-fries and veggie burgers. Serve these dishes with appealing side dishes. A green salad and crusty bread taste great with lasagna, while rice and pineapple chunks complement a stir-fry, and coleslaw and brownies go well with veggie burgers.

❖ Unite complementary foods. Soup with sandwiches or salad is a perfect example. Baked potatoes with salad is another idea. Be sure to keep the foods interesting. For example, when you choose baked potatoes and salad, serve the potatoes loaded with toppings such as salsa and black beans or tomato sauce and mozzarella cheese, and make the salad extra special with the additions of fruits, seeds, legumes and grains.

❖ Think ethnic. Ethiopian, Thai, Italian, Mexican, Japanese, Indian—all of these cuisines have ample vegetarian dishes. With most of the world eating a primarily vegetarian diet, it's no wonder that their cuisines would play up the splendor of grains, vegetables, fruits and legumes. So delight in *pasta e fagioli* (macaroni and beans), curries, *tabouli* (bulgur salad), risotto (an Italian dish made with arborio rice), burritos, chop suey and other dishes from around the world. Serve side dishes that support the entrée. That means rice, chutney and raita with curries, seasoned grains and refried beans with burritos and rice with chop suey.

❖ Eat breakfast for dinner. Try waffles with fresh berries, blintzes, potato pancakes with applesauce, and oatmeal topped with fruit. These kid pleasers are tops in vitamins and minerals.

❖ Load up on legumes. The humble bean has been all but forgotten in the average American diet, but this nutrient- and fiber-packed food is too good to pass up. Bean soups warm up a chilly day, and bean-studded salad turns lettuce into a substantial meal. Serve both types of meals with breadsticks, rolls or other breadstuff plus fruit. Also combine beans with grains. Dishes like hoppin' John (black-eyed peas with rice) and bean tacos (the corn-based taco is the grain) are downright satisfying. Serve hoppin' John with greens and tacos with the trimmings (shredded lettuce and tomato) and sliced oranges.

❖ Incorporate soy foods into your meals. With dozens of scientific studies touting the health benefits of soy (see "It's Soy Good," page 82), it's time to discover this Asian delight. Foods like tofu, tempeh, textured vegetable protein and soy milk can be added to dishes in many ways. Tofu or tempeh, for instance, may be cubed, skewered along with vegetables and grilled. You can also blend tofu with other ingredients to make flavorful dips. Textured vegetable protein can take the place of ground beef in saucy recipes. Soy milk may replace cow's milk in baked goods or be poured over breakfast cereal.

❖ Don't forget dessert. Dessert need not be a nutrition no-no. By choosing low-fat desserts, many of which will be heavy on fruit (think baked apples, fruit crumbles, rice pudding with raisins), you can add nutrition to the meal—and a lot of satisfaction.

THE FAMILY DINNER

Now that you have a sense of meal making, you ought to know something else: While trend surveys indicate that fewer families are eating dinner together regularly, health research suggests that sharing meals is good for digestion *and* forging strong familial bonds.

Whatever's to blame—television, kids' after-school activities, busy work schedules, long commutes—it's clear that children learn a great deal about the world while sitting around the dinner table. They learn sharing, the art of conversation, good manners and respect for other people. They also learn about good nutrition.

The family dinner table is a powerful symbol of togetherness. It may be the only place during the day when the entire family joins hands, figuratively or literally. It's a gateway to finding meaning in relationships—to food, yes, but most important, to our children and each other.

One last thing: When you sit down to eat, unplug the phone or turn on the answering machine. You'll be glad you shut out the world, if only for a little while.

KEEP IN BALANCE

For the most exciting meals, vary colors, textures (crunchy, smooth, chewy) and flavors (sweet, sour, pungent, bland). A meal of fettucini alfredo, cauliflower and rice pudding is boring (very white, very bland), while lentil-barley soup with crusty bread and sliced fruit is sure to please.

Also consider the season. A pasta salad works well on an August afternoon, but shepherd's pie makes sense in winter. And balance the entire meal: If the main dish and side dishes are heavy, select a light dessert. But if dinner is a beautiful but light salad with breadsticks, why not serve cake?

Truly, the best meals are balanced in every way—nutrition, color, flavor and season.

Thirty Family Menu Ideas

1. Italian Spaghetti Pie (p. 166)
   green salad
   Three-Fruit Kebabs (p. 194)

2. Vegetable Curry with Basmati Rice (p. 183)
   Cool Cucumber Raita (p. 194)
   chutney

3. Broccoli Stir-Fry in Sweet-Sour Sauce (p. 168)
   brown rice
   chunks of pineapple

4. Skinny Shepherd's Pie (p. 185)
   Banana-ana Bread (p. 202)

5. Black Bean Chili (p. 184)
   corn bread
   green salad

6. Confetti Pasta Salad with Vinaigrette (use the variation) (p. 162)
   Apple Streusel Cake (p. 201)

7. Vegetable Kebabs (p. 170)
   brown rice or wild rice
   sliced bananas

8. Sloppy Joeys (p. 188)
   Apple Coleslaw (p. 161)
   Oatmeal Chocolate Chip Cookies (p. 206)

9. Sunburst Burgers (p. 186)
   Carrot Salad with Orange and Raisins (p. 160)
   oven-baked french fries

10. Lentil-Barley Soup (p. 157)
    crusty bread
    apple slices

11. Creamy Broccoli Soup (p. 158)
    Lasagna in a Blanket (p. 165)
    pear slices

12. Lots-of-Vegetables Pizza (p. 163)
    Fruit Juice Pops (p. 208)

13. Pineapple-Peanut Bow Ties (p. 186)
    Orange-Apple-Raisin Salad (p. 158)

14. Lean Bean Burritos (p. 177)
    Spanish Rice (p. 193)
    Carrot Mini-Muffins (p. 204)

15. Apricot and Bulgur Stuffed Crepes (p. 182)
    Brown Gravy (p. 198)
    Chocolate Brownie Cake (p. 199)

16. Cheesy Potato Pancakes (p. 175)
    Raspberry Applesauce (p. 195)
    nonfat sour cream

17. Savory 'n' Sweet Rice (p. 176)
    steamed broccoli or green beans
    sliced peaches

18. Alphabet Vegetable Soup (p. 156)
    crusty bread or crackers
    Silly Spider Cookies (p. 208)

19. Bean Stew with Vegetables and Couscous (p. 171)
    green salad
    Cinnamon-Raisin Bread Pudding (p. 205)

20. Green Peppers Stuffed with Basmati Rice and Chickpeas (p. 180)
    steamed carrots
    Cookie-Cutter Cookies (p. 207)

21. Lentil-Tomato Mostaccioli (p. 167)
    green salad
    Spinach-Ricotta Dip with crackers (p. 156)

22. Low-Fat Cheesy Spinach Squares (p. 173)
    whole-wheat rolls
    sliced cantaloupe

23. Casserole Olé (p. 178)
    orange slices
    Oatmeal-Raisin Cookies (p. 206)

24. Bean and Spinach Cassoulet (p. 179)
    Sour Cream Whipped Potatoes (p. 191)
    apple slices

25. Low-Fat PB&J (p. 190)
    Stuffed Celery with Raisins (p. 154)
    red and green grapes

26. Great Bean Lunch Spread (p. 189)
    whole-grain bread slices
    Low-Fat Potato Salad (p. 159)
    Oatmeal Chocolate Chip Cookies (p. 206)

27. Savory Baked Samosas (p. 181)
    brown rice
    Cool Cucumber Raita (p. 194)

28. Simple Pita Pizza (p. 164)
    raw vegetables
    Carrot Mini-Muffins (p. 204)

29. Nachos Muchachos (p. 155)
    Lean Bean Tacos (p. 177)
    chunks of watermelon

30. Tempeh and Broccoli Stir-Fry in Teriyaki Sauce (p. 168)
    brown rice
    Ambrosia (p. 205)

WHAT IS IT?

The following glossary reflects the ingredients called for in the recipes. Some of them may be unfamiliar to you; others may be an integral part of your cooking, but I've included them to share extra information. You can find these ingredients in well-stocked supermarkets and natural food stores.

CILANTRO
This zesty-flavored herb comes from the coriander plant. Fresh cilantro is far more flavorful than dried, so use fresh whenever possible. It's common in Indian and Hispanic cuisines.

EGG REPLACER
The common egg replacer contains egg whites and other ingredients that produce a product that closely mimics whole eggs. You can use egg replacer in baked goods and to make omelets and other egg dishes. Its big advantage is the lack of cholesterol. If you want an eggless egg replacer, count on a trip to a natural food store, where you can buy a product that provides the leavening and binding properties of eggs. The eggless replacer cannot be used to make egg dishes.

FLOURS
Whole-wheat flour. More flavorful than white flour, whole-wheat flour is rich in protein, many vitamins including B vitamins (except B_{12}) and fiber. It's the best choice for bread baking. Store whole-wheat flour in your refrigerator or freezer to prevent rancidity.
Whole-wheat pastry flour. Milled from lower-protein wheat, whole-wheat pastry flour makes tender baked goods. Other than protein content, this flour has a nutritional profile similar to that of regular whole-wheat flour. Store in your refrigerator or freezer.
Unbleached white flour. This flour has half the calcium and one-fourth the iron, phosphorus, potassium and B vitamins of whole-wheat flour. Yet it's a better choice than bleached flour, which is more refined.

GINGERROOT
The grayish, knobby rootstock of the ginger plant is now common in supermarket produce sections. Grate or slice it to add zing to dishes. Store gingerroot in your refrigerator or freezer.

GRAINS
Barley. Chewy and delicately flavored, this grain comes in two types—unrefined whole barley, sometimes called pot barley, and refined barley, or pearl barley, which has had its hard outer layers removed. The latter has less fiber and fewer nutrients than unrefined whole barley.
Basmati rice. This quick-cooking grain is fragrant and nutty. It's traditional in Indian cooking but works well in a variety of dishes.
Brown rice. This unrefined rice is nutritionally superior to white rice, which has been stripped of its bran and polished. Though some white rice is enriched, it has no potassium, compared to the 137 milligrams in one cup cooked brown rice, and only 31 milligrams of phosphorus, compared to the 142 milligrams in one cup cooked brown rice. Brown rice is also far richer in fiber. It's available in three types: short, medium and long. Short-grain brown rice is the sweetest and is the best choice for desserts like rice pudding; the longer varieties make great pilafs, salads and casseroles.
Bulgur. Sometimes called bulgur wheat or cracked wheat, this quick-cooking grain has a wonderfully nutty flavor that works well in many dishes.
Couscous. Technically, couscous is a pasta, but most people think it's a grain because it soaks up water like other grains and becomes fluffy when gently stirred with a fork. It cooks quickly and has a delicate flavor.
Rolled oats. These are the type used to make oatmeal. Rich in fiber and tops in taste, they may be incorporated into many dishes, including veggie burgers and baked goods.

RASPBERRY VINEGAR
Sweet and sassy, this vinegar adds a fruity flavor to dressings, marinades and other dishes. Other flavored vinegars are also on the market.

SOY FOODS
Examples are soybeans, soy milk, soy yogurt, soy sauce, tamari, tempeh, tofu, textured vegetable protein. See page 82 for details.

VEGETABLE OILS
The healthiest types are canola, olive and safflower. These three types are preferred because they are higher in monounsaturated fats than are other vegetable oils. No matter which you choose, use a light hand with oil in your cooking: Fat is fat.

VEGETARIAN WORCESTERSHIRE SAUCE
With a flavor identical to traditional Worcestershire sauce, this product omits anchovies. Look for it in natural food stores.

WHITE BUTTON MUSHROOMS
These are the type readily found in supermarkets. Wipe them clean before using. When you're in an adventuresome mood, substitute wild mushrooms for white button mushrooms.

ABOUT THE NUTRITIONAL BREAKDOWNS

I've provided nutritional breakdowns to aid you in planning meals. My hope is that you'll develop a general awareness of the nutrition of foods so you can apply your new knowledge to your family's diet and replace your high-fat, high-cholesterol, high-sodium recipes with healthful choices.

Please resist the temptation to eat by numbers. That spoils the fun of dining. And vegetarian meals ought to be celebratory.

Instead, apply the *principles* of healthful eating to your diet and let the numbers of the nutritional breakdowns fall where they may. They're bound to reflect good nutrition when you choose good foods to eat.

That said, here's an explanation of the nutritional breakdowns. Using a software program that calculates calories, protein, fat and so on, I figured in all of the ingredients listed in each recipe, except when an ingredient is optional. In this case, I omitted it from the breakdown. When a choice of ingredients is given (such as ¼ to ½ cup sliced carrots, or 1 tablespoon margarine or butter), I used the first number or food listed. Where the quantity is unspecified, such as "Salt to taste," I chose a reasonable amount.

Because the healthfulness of one's diet is reflected over a day or days of meals, my nutritional breakdowns do not provide percentages of calories from fat. I believe it's fine to eat a higher-fat dish if the bulk of the diet is low in fat. The same goes with other nutrients.

The road to healthful eating is balance and good taste. The nutritional breakdowns are an aid to that end. To your health and culinary enjoyment, I wish you the finest.

Key

CAL.: calories	CARB.: carbohydrates	FIBER: total dietary fiber
PROT.: protein	CHOL.: cholesterol	G: gram
FAT: total fat	SOD.: sodium	MG: milligram

10

Beginnings

These appetizers, soups and salads make a great start to a meal. When your family isn't too hungry, many of these recipes can *be* the meal—ideally a lunch or a simple supper—with the addition of crusty bread and some fruit.

Stuffed Celery with Raisins

This crunchy and not-too-sweet appetizer also makes a great kid's lunch. It's rich in fiber, protein, calcium and iron.

4 stalks celery

⅓ cup nut butter (such as peanut or almond)

⅓ cup reduced-fat tofu or nonfat cream cheese

1 teaspoon honey or maple syrup

½ cup raisins

Cut the stalks crosswise. Combine the nut butter, tofu or cream cheese and honey or maple syrup. Spread this mixture into the cavity of the celery. Push the raisins into the nut butter mixture. Serve.

Serves 8.

PER SERVING: 103 CAL.; 4G PROT.; 5G FAT; 11G CARB.; 0 CHOL.; 26MG SOD.; 1.7G FIBER.

Nachos Muchachos

This low-fat snack has a mild Mexican flavor.

4 cups baked tortilla chips

⅓ cup nonfat sour cream

1 cup shredded reduced-fat cheddar cheese

1 4-ounce can minced green chilies

2 fresh plum tomatoes, diced

¾ cup cooked red kidney beans

Preheat the broiler. Place the tortilla chips in a single layer on the bottom of a large baking pan. In a small bowl, mix together the sour cream, cheese and chilies. Spread this mixture on the tortilla chips, covering them completely. Sprinkle the tomatoes and red beans on top. Broil until the cheese melts, about 3 minutes. Watch carefully to avoid burning. Transfer to a platter and serve warm.

Serves 8.

PER SERVING: 112 CAL.; 8G PROT.; 3G FAT; 14G CARB.; 10MG CHOL.; 326MG SOD.; 2G FIBER.

Season with Care

Adding too much seasoning to a dish is worse than adding too little. In the latter scenario, you still have an opportunity to enhance your creation with salt, herbs and spices to make it just right. But if you're heavy on the seasonings, a culinary rescue may be impossible. So when seasoning your dishes, proceed with care.

Spinach-Ricotta Dip

Scoop up this creamy dip, which is far lower in fat than regular dips, with whole-grain crackers or raw vegetables. It's a fun way to eat nutrient-packed spinach.

1 10-ounce package frozen chopped spinach, thawed and squeezed dry

¾ cup part-skim ricotta cheese

¾ cup nonfat sour cream

1 clove garlic, minced (optional)

2 scallions (green and white parts), sliced

1 tablespoon fresh dill or 1 teaspoon dried

Salt and freshly ground black pepper to taste

In a blender or food processor or with a fork, thoroughly combine the spinach, ricotta and sour cream. Transfer this mixture to a serving bowl. Gently stir in the remaining ingredients. Chill.

VARIATION:

Add 1 to 2 diced fresh plum tomatoes to the dip before serving.

Makes 2 cups; 16 2-tablespoon servings.

PER SERVING: 32 CAL.; 3G PROT.; 1G FAT; 3G CARB.; 4MG CHOL.; 76MG SOD.; 0.6G FIBER.

Alphabet Vegetable Soup

Here's alphabet soup at its finest: a wonderful aroma, great taste and exceptional nutrition.

½ onion, sliced

2 carrots, sliced

1 stalk celery, sliced

2 potatoes, peeled and cubed

1 cup green beans

1 28-ounce can diced tomatoes, with juice

8 cups vegetable stock or 8 cups water with 1 vegetable bouillon cube

6 ounces uncooked alphabet pasta

Salt and freshly ground black pepper to taste

In a large pot, combine the onion, carrots, celery, potatoes, green beans, tomatoes with juice and vegetable stock or water and bouillon cube. Bring to a boil, reduce the heat and let simmer until the vegetables are tender, about 30 minutes. Add the pasta and cook until al dente, about 8 minutes. Season with the salt and pepper. Serve warm.

VARIATIONS:

❖ Replace the alphabet pasta with any small pasta.

❖ Use leftover cooked pasta in place of uncooked pasta. Add it to the pot 5 minutes before serving to warm through.
❖ Add 1 cup of your favorite cooked legumes: navy beans, red kidney beans, black beans.

Serves 6.

PER SERVING: 200 CAL.; 7G PROT.; 0.6G FAT; 42G CARB.; 0 CHOL.; 384MG SOD.; 6.4G FIBER

Lentil-Barley Soup

A bowlful of this soup provides protein and nutrients—and warms up tummies on chilly days.

6 cups vegetable stock or 6 cups water with 1 vegetable bouillon cube

1 cup uncooked brown lentils

½ cup uncooked barley

1 stalk celery, sliced

1 carrot, sliced

2 fresh plum tomatoes, quartered and sliced

½ onion or 3 scallions (green and white parts), sliced

¼ teaspoon ground cumin

½ to 1 teaspoon fresh cilantro

1 clove garlic, minced

In a large pot, place all the ingredients, cover and bring to a boil. Reduce the heat and simmer, covered. Let cook for 1 hour. Serve warm.

Serves 6.

PER SERVING: 183 CAL.; 10G PROT.; 1G FAT; 36G CARB.; 0 CHOL.; 18MG SOD.; 10G FIBER.

Creamy Broccoli Soup

A creamy soup with no cream? That's right. The secret is pureed potatoes, which add extra nutrients to the soup without a smidgeon of fat.

2 cups chopped fresh broccoli

3½ cups vegetable stock or 3 ½ cups water with 1 vegetable bouillon cube

4 potatoes, peeled and cubed

½ onion, chopped

½ to 1 tablespoon fresh cilantro

Salt and freshly ground black pepper to taste

Place all the ingredients except the salt and pepper and ½ cup vegetable stock or water in a large pot. Bring to a boil, cover and cook over medium heat until tender, about 20 minutes. Set aside ½ cup broccoli to use as a garnish.

Puree the remaining contents of the pot, a batch at a time, in a blender or food processor. Be sure to fill the blender or food processor no more than ⅔ full. Return the pureed soup to the pot. Add the remaining vegetable stock or water, season with the salt and pepper and simmer 5 minutes. Pour the soup into individual bowls and top each one with the reserved broccoli garnish. Serve warm.

Serves 6.

PER SERVING: 91 CAL.; 3G PROT.; 0.2G FAT; 21G CARB.; 0 CHOL.; 368MG SOD.; 2.7G FIBER.

Orange-Apple-Raisin Salad

This colorful salad may accompany a main dish or be served at the end of a meal as dessert.

2 seedless oranges, white pith removed

1 Rome Beauty or other sweet red apple

½ cup raisins

1 stalk celery, sliced

1 tablespoon packed brown sugar

1 tablespoon fresh lemon juice

Cut the oranges and apple into bite-size pieces. Combine them in a medium bowl with the remaining ingredients. Chill.

Serves 4.

PER SERVING: 141 CAL.; 1G PROT.; 1G FAT; 36G CARB.; 0 CHOL.; 12MG SOD.; 4.6G FIBER.

Low-Fat Potato Salad

10 potatoes, washed

Water to cover

2 to 3 hard-boiled eggs

2 stalks celery, sliced

1 green or red bell pepper, cored and chopped

⅓ cup nonfat sour cream

⅓ cup low-fat or fat-free mayonnaise

½ teaspoon salt or to taste

In a large pot, bring the potatoes to a gentle boil in water and let cook until fork-tender, about 20 to 30 minutes. Drain. Refrigerate until thoroughly chilled.

Peel the potatoes. Discard the peelings. Cut the potatoes into chunks and place them in a large bowl. Peel and mince the eggs. Add them to the bowl along with the celery and bell pepper. In a small bowl, combine the sour cream and mayonnaise. Stir into the potato mixture, coating all of the vegetables. Season with the salt. Cover and chill.

VARIATION:

Add 1 teaspoon Dijon-style mustard, 2 teaspoons pickle relish or 1 tablespoon fresh herbs to the sour cream and mayonnaise mixture before combining with the potato mixture.

Serves 8.

PER SERVING: 211 CAL.; 6G PROT.; 4G FAT; 38G CARB.; 53MG CHOL.; 260MG SOD.; 3.4G FIBER.

Succotash Salad

1 10-ounce package frozen lima beans, rinsed

1 cup whole-kernel corn

1 scallion (green and white parts), sliced

½ cup fat-free red wine salad dressing or your favorite vinaigrette

Diced tomato for garnish

Cook the lima beans according to package directions. Let cool.

Combine the lima beans, corn, scallion and dressing in a medium bowl. Let sit, covered, in the refrigerator for at least 1 hour, stirring occasionally. Garnish with the tomato.

Serves 4.

PER SERVING: 129 CAL.; 6G PROT.; 0.4G FAT, 26G CARB.; 0 CHOL.; 544MG SOD.; 4.4G FIBER.

Carrot Salad with Orange and Raisins

Serve this naturally sweet salad with dollops of yogurt if desired.

½ pound carrots, shredded

1 seedless orange, white pith removed, cut into bite-size pieces

¼ cup raisins

1 tablespoon safflower or canola oil

1½ to 2 tablespoons raspberry vinegar or rice wine vinegar

½ teaspoon fresh cilantro

Salt to taste

In a serving dish, combine the carrots, orange and raisins. In a small bowl, whisk together the remaining ingredients and pour over the carrot mixture; toss. Chill.

Serves 4.

PER SERVING: 97 CAL.; 1G PROT.; 4G FAT; 17G CARB.; 0 CHOL.; 154MG SOD.; 2.9G FIBER.

Apple Coleslaw

Apple slices add a refreshing touch to this coleslaw. Let it chill for a couple of hours before serving so flavors can meld.

½ small head green cabbage, cored and finely shredded

2 carrots, finely shredded

1 Rome Beauty or other sweet apple, cored and sliced

1 to 2 tablespoons diced onion

2 tablespoons red wine vinegar

1 tablespoon virgin olive oil

2 teaspoons Dijon-style mustard

2 teaspoons sugar

½ teaspoon celery seeds

Salt and freshly ground black pepper to taste

Chopped fresh parsley for garnish

In a large bowl, combine the cabbage, carrots, apple and onion. In a small bowl, whisk together the remaining ingredients except the parsley. Pour over the cabbage mixture and toss. Garnish with the parsley. Chill.

Serves 4.

PER SERVING: 87 CAL.; 1G PROT.; 4G FAT; 13G CARB.; 0 CHOL.; 218MG SOD.; 2.6G FIBER.

Confetti Pasta Salad with Vinaigrette

Small pasta teams with a slew of vegetables to make a flavorful salad that's perfect alongside a main dish or on its own.

SALAD

- 6 ounces uncooked tiny shell or bow-tie pasta
- 1 2 ¼-ounce can sliced black olives, rinsed
- 1 cup frozen peas, thawed under cool running water
- 2 carrots, thinly sliced
- 1 fresh plum tomato, diced
- ¾ cup whole-kernel corn
- ¼ to ½ cup shredded part-skim mozzarella or reduced-fat cheddar cheese (optional)

DRESSING

- 3 tablespoons raspberry vinegar or rice wine vinegar
- 2 tablespoons virgin olive oil
- 1 clove garlic, minced
- 1 scallion (green and white parts), sliced

- ½ teaspoon dried oregano
- ½ teaspoon dried basil
- Salt and freshly ground black pepper to taste

Salad: Cook the pasta according to package directions. Drain and rinse under cool running water; drain. Place the pasta in a serving bowl. Combine with the remaining salad ingredients.

Dressing: Whisk together the dressing ingredients. Pour over the salad and toss. Chill.

VARIATION:

For a more substantial salad, add 1 cup cooked red kidney beans or other favorite legume.

Serves 8.

PER SERVING: 168 CAL.; 5G PROT.; 5G FAT; 27G CARB.; 0 CHOL.; 175MG SOD.; 3.4G FIBER.

11

Middles

All of these main dishes and side dishes are family-friendly, and some are healthful revisions of traditionally high-fat recipes. They represent a variety of cuisines, including Mexican, Italian, Chinese, Indian and American. Be sure to update your recipe file with these winners.

Lots-of-Vegetables Pizza

Vary the vegetables to suit the taste of your family. Here's one well-loved version.

1 tomato, thinly sliced

1 12-inch prepared pizza crust

2 teaspoons virgin olive oil

½ onion, thinly sliced

8 white button mushrooms, chopped

1 green bell pepper, cored and chopped

1 tablespoon fresh oregano or 1 teaspoon dried

1 cup shredded part-skim mozzarella cheese

Preheat the oven to 375 degrees. Arrange the tomato slices on the pizza crust. Set aside. In a medium pan over medium-high heat, heat the olive oil and sauté the onion, mushrooms and green pepper until softened, about 5 minutes. Sprinkle the vegetables and oregano over the tomato slices. Top with the mozzarella. Bake 15 to 20 minutes. Slice and serve warm.

Serves 4.

PER SERVING: 281 CAL.; 13G PROT.; 7G FAT; 42G CARB.; 10MG CHOL.; 589MG SOD.; 2.7G FIBER.

Simple Pita Pizza

These mini-pizzas take only minutes to prepare and cook.

- 4 6-inch pita rounds
- ½ cup Chunky Tomato Sauce (see recipe, page 197) or your favorite store-bought tomato sauce
- 1 cup shredded part-skim mozzarella cheese

Preheat the oven to 400 degrees. Place the pita rounds on a cookie sheet. Top each pita round with 2 tablespoons of tomato sauce and ¼ cup cheese. Bake until the cheese is bubbly, about 10 minutes. Let cool slightly before serving.

VARIATION:

Before adding the cheese, top the pita rounds with cubed tofu or sliced tofu hot dogs.

Serves 4.

PER SERVING: 235 CAL.; 14G PROT.; 5G FAT; 34G CARB.; 10MG CHOL.; 675MG SOD.; 4.5G FIBER.

Spinach Surprise

I've called for frozen spinach in these recipes for several reasons. Ease of preparation tops the list. Busy moms and dads can rarely find time to meticulously wash, trim, cook and chop bunches of spinach. What's better, spinach suffers no nutritive value in freezing, and frozen spinach tastes almost identical to fresh spinach after cooking. Packages of frozen chopped spinach are widely available in the freezer section of your supermarket.

If you prefer fresh spinach, use about ¾ pound fresh spinach to equal the amount in 1 10-ounce package of frozen chopped spinach. After trimming the fresh spinach, rinse it thoroughly. Then, with the water still clinging to it, place it in a large, dry saucepan and wilt it over medium heat for about 3 minutes. Rinse under cool water, squeeze dry and chop.

Lasagna in a Blanket

This combination of pasta, tomato sauce, cheese and spinach is a kid's fa-vorite. Even ''spinach haters'' usually like it.

8 uncooked lasagna noodles

1 to 2 teaspoons virgin olive oil

1 to 2 cloves garlic, minced

½ onion, chopped

1 10-ounce package frozen chopped spinach, thawed and squeezed dry

1 cup part-skim ricotta cheese or low-fat cottage cheese (see note)

Dash nutmeg

Salt and freshly ground black pepper to taste

2 cups thick tomato sauce

1 tablespoon fresh basil or 1 teaspoon dried

¼ to ½ cup shredded part-skim mozzarella cheese (optional)

Cook the noodles in boiling wa-ter until barely tender. Rinse and let stand in cool water while preparing the spinach-cheese mixture.

In a large pan over medium heat, heat the oil and sauté the garlic and onion until the onion is transparent, about 7 minutes. Remove from the heat. To the pan, add the spinach, ricotta or cottage cheese, nutmeg, salt and pepper. Combine thoroughly. Coat each noodle with about 3 tablespoons of the spinach-cheese mixture along its entire length. Then roll up the noodles and place them seam side down in a 13 × 9-inch baking pan.

Pour the tomato sauce over the rolled-up noodles, covering them completely, and sprinkle with the basil and mozzarella if desired. Bake, uncovered, until heated through, about 20 to 25 minutes.

NOTE: Cottage cheese is a nice alternative to ricotta, but the lat-ter gives a more authentic taste.

Serves 4.

PER SERVING: 365 CAL.; 20G PROT.; 8G FAT; 52G CARB.; 22MG CHOL.; 917MG SOD.; 6.4G FIBER.

Italian Spaghetti Pie

This is a tasty dish to use up leftover spaghetti. Be sure to heat the cooked spaghetti in a microwave oven or with a quick dunk in boiling water before adding the olive oil.

6 ounces spaghetti, cooked and drained

1 tablespoon virgin olive oil

½ onion, sliced

2 eggs, lightly beaten, or equivalent egg substitute

2 to 4 tablespoons grated Parmesan cheese, preferably fresh

1 cup part-skim ricotta cheese

1 cup Chunky Tomato Sauce (see recipe, page 197) or your favorite store-bought tomato sauce

¼ to ½ cup shredded part-skim mozzarella cheese

2 teaspoons fresh oregano or ½ teaspoon dried

In a medium bowl, toss the hot spaghetti with 2 teaspoons of the olive oil. Set aside. In a medium pan over medium-high heat, heat the remaining olive oil and sauté the onion until barely transparent, about 5 minutes. Set aside.

Preheat the oven to 350 degrees. Lightly grease a 9-inch pie plate. Set aside. Add the eggs or egg substitute and Parmesan to the spaghetti and stir to combine. Pour into the pie plate. Spread the ricotta on top. Completely cover the ricotta and spaghetti with the tomato sauce. Sprinkle the mozzarella and oregano on top. Bake, uncovered, for 25 to 30 minutes. Let cool 5 minutes before cutting into wedges.

Serves 4.

PER SERVING: 349 CAL.; 18G PROT.; 13G FAT; 38G CARB.; 130MG CHOL.; 447MG SOD.; 2.3G FIBER.

Lentil-Tomato Mostaccioli

This pasta dish is made extra special and satisfying with the addition of lentils. You may replace the mostaccioli (tubular pasta) with other favorite noodle shapes, such as linguine, radiatore (pasta nuggets) or shells.

12 ounces uncooked mostaccioli

 2 cups Chunky Tomato Sauce (see recipe, page 197) or your favorite store-bought tomato sauce

¾ to 1 cup cooked brown lentils

½ cup shredded part-skim mozzarella cheese (optional)

Fresh parsley, oregano or basil for garnish

Cook the pasta according to package directions; drain. Transfer to an ovenproof serving dish. In a saucepan over medium heat, warm the tomato sauce and lentils. Spoon over the mostaccioli. Top with the mozzarella cheese if desired and heat in a broiler until the cheese melts, about 3 minutes. Garnish with the fresh herbs.

Serves 6.

PER SERVING: 299 CAL.; 12G PROT.; 1G FAT; 59G CARB.; 0 CHOL.; 611MG SOD.; 4.5G FIBER.

Broccoli Stir-Fry in Sweet-Sour Sauce

This next-to-no-fat dish is sweetened by juice and has a slew of vitamin-rich vegetables. If your younger children don't like sauces, spoon out some of the cooked vegetables onto their dishes before adding the sweet-sour sauce to the skillet.

½ teaspoon safflower or canola oil

½ onion, sliced

1 clove garlic, minced

1 1-pound bag frozen stir-fry vegetables with broccoli

1 tablespoon soy sauce or tamari

¾ cup pineapple juice

2 to 3 tablespoons red wine vinegar

1 teaspoon cornstarch dissolved in 1 tablespoon water

3 cups cooked brown rice

In a large skillet over medium-high heat, heat the oil and sauté the onion and garlic until barely softened, about 3 to 5 minutes. Add the frozen vegetables, reduce the heat to medium and cover. Stir the vegetables every few minutes until they're warmed through, about 10 minutes. Uncover the skillet.

Combine the soy sauce or tamari, pineapple juice and vinegar in a small bowl. Stir into the vegetables. When the liquid starts to simmer, stir in the dissolved cornstarch. Continue to stir until the sauce thickens. Remove from the heat.

Divide the rice among 4 plates. Spoon the stir-fry on top or to the side. Serve.

VARIATIONS:

❖ Add leftover vegetables to the stir-fry when the vegetables are no longer frozen.

❖ For TOFU AND BROCCOLI STIR-FRY IN SWEET-SOUR SAUCE, cut ½ pound of firm tofu into ½-inch cubes. Sauté in 1 to 2 teaspoons of safflower or canola oil until lightly browned. Gently stir the sautéed tofu into the stir-fry once the sauce thickens.

❖ For TEMPEH AND BROCCOLI STIR-FRY IN TERIYAKI SAUCE, add ½ pound sliced tempeh to the skillet with the stir-fry vegetables. Omit the soy sauce, pineapple juice and red wine vinegar and replace with 1 cup bottled teriyaki sauce. Proceed with the recipe.

Serves 4.

PER SERVING: 250 CAL.; 7G PROT.; 2G FAT; 52G CARB.; 0 CHOL.; 284MG SOD.; 6.4G FIBER.

Grains Cookery

Cooking grains is easy. You simply put a pot of grains and liquid to simmer on the stove and let the steam do the work while you putter around the kitchen finishing other cooking tasks.

You may choose the boiling water method or the cold water method to cook grains. For the boiling water method, bring a pot of water or vegetable broth to a boil and sprinkle in the grain. Cover the pot with a tight-fitting lid and simmer. This method causes the grain to swell quickly and keeps the grains separate. For the cold water method, place the grain in a pot, add cold water, cover with a tight-fitting lid and bring to a boil, then simmer.

Simmering (covered)

GRAIN	WATER PER CUP OF DRY GRAIN	COOKING TIME	YIELD (APPROX.)
Whole barley (presoaked)	2½ to 3 cups	1 hour	3 cups
Bulgur	1½ cups	15 minutes	2½ cups
Corn grits	4 cups	15 minutes	3 to 4 cups
Couscous			
Whole grain	2 cups	5 minutes	4 cups
Refined	1½ cups	5 minutes	4 cups
Kasha	1¾ cups	30 minutes	4 cups
Millet	2 cups	30 minutes	3 to 4 cups
Brown rice	1¾ cups	45 minutes	3 to 4 cups
Quinoa	1½ cups	15 minutes	4 cups
Teff	3 cups	15 minutes	3 cups
Wild rice	2½ cups	35 minutes	3 cups

Vegetable Kebabs

Kids love to thread skewers with colorful vegetables. Let them stir together the marinade too, under your supervision.

KEBABS

- 12 medium white button mushrooms
- 2 green bell peppers, cored and cut into 12 large pieces
- 1 stalk broccoli, cut into 12 large florets
- 12 small new potatoes, whole, or 4 small baking potatoes, quartered
- 12 cherry tomatoes

MARINADE

- 4 tablespoons fresh lemon juice
- 4 tablespoons red wine vinegar
- 2 tablespoons virgin olive oil
- 1 clove garlic, minced
- 1 scallion (green and white parts), minced
- 4 cups cooked brown rice

Kebabs: In a saucepan fitted with a steamer basket, steam the mushrooms, peppers and broccoli until barely tender, about 4 minutes. Set aside. Steam the potatoes until barely tender, about 15 minutes. Let cool slightly. Skewer the vegetables and the cherry tomatoes on 6 skewers, alternating the vegetables, until each skewer has 2 of each kind of vegetable. Set aside.

Marinade: In a large, shallow pan, stir together the marinade ingredients. Place the skewers in the marinade and let stand at least 30 minutes, turning the skewers occasionally. Grill or broil, turning the kebabs and brushing with the marinade until lightly browned, about 5 to 10 minutes.

Divide the rice among 6 plates. Slip the vegetables off the skewers and onto the rice. Serve warm.

VARIATION:

For VEGETABLE AND TOFU KE-BABS, freeze ½ pound of firm tofu and let thaw. Drain thoroughly. Cut the tofu into 12 cubes. Place on the skewers with the vegetables and proceed with the recipe.

Serves 6.

PER SERVING: 255 CAL.; 7G PROT.; 4G FAT; 49G CARB.; 0 CHOL.; 208MG SOD.; 7.8G FIBER.

Bean Stew with Vegetables and Couscous

Couscous adds extra body to this flavorful stew.

1 16-ounce can kidney beans, rinsed

1 16-ounce can chickpeas, rinsed

1 medium onion, cut in half and sliced thinly

1 clove garlic, minced

1 teaspoon dried oregano, crumbled

1 tablespoon chili powder

Dash salt and freshly ground black pepper

¼ teaspoon cayenne pepper or to taste

2 medium carrots, thinly sliced on the diagonal

1 green or red bell pepper, cored and chopped

½ cup whole-kernel corn or other vegetable of your choice

1 28-ounce can diced tomatoes

1 cup uncooked couscous

Combine all the ingredients except the couscous in a medium pot and cook over medium heat until the vegetables soften, about 30 minutes. Stir in the couscous, cover and remove from the heat. Let sit 5 to 10 minutes before serving.

Serves 4.

PER SERVING: 543 CAL.; 23G PROT.; 3G FAT; 112G CARB.; 0 CHOL.; 628MG SOD.; 16G FIBER.

Spinach-Rice Casserole

For kids who aren't keen on casseroles, spoon portions of the brown rice, tomatoes and cheese onto their plates before combining the ingredients. This dish tastes great as is or topped with your favorite tomato sauce.

4 cups cooked brown rice

2 10-ounce packages frozen chopped spinach, thawed and squeezed dry

4 fresh plum tomatoes, chopped, or 1 cup salsa

2 scallions (green and white parts), chopped

2 to 4 teaspoons soy sauce or tamari

4 to 6 ounces shredded reduced-fat cheddar or Monterey Jack cheese

2 eggs, lightly beaten, or equivalent egg substitute

Preheat the oven to 350 degrees. In a large bowl, thoroughly com-bine all the ingredients. Spoon into a lightly greased 2-quart casserole dish. Bake until firm, about 35 to 45 minutes. Let cool slightly and serve.

VARIATIONS:

❖ Omit the cheese and eggs and add 1 or 2 tablespoons toasted sunflower seeds or nuts of your choice.
❖ Stir in 1 tablespoon chopped fresh herbs, such as basil or ci-lantro, before heating.

Serves 6.

PER SERVING: 276 CAL.; 15G PROT.; 7G FAT; 40G CARB.; 84MG CHOL.; 355MG SOD.; 6.2G FIBER.

Low-Fat Cheesy Spinach Squares

This entrée of spinach and low-fat cheeses makes a beta-carotene- and calcium-rich dinner or brunch.

1 teaspoon butter

½ onion, sliced

3 cups low-fat cottage cheese

4 eggs, lightly beaten

2 10-ounce packages frozen chopped spinach, thawed and squeezed dry

¼ to ½ cup shredded reduced-fat cheddar cheese

Salt to taste

In a small nonstick skillet over medium-low heat, melt the butter. Add the onion, stirring frequently, until the onion is transparent, about 7 minutes.

Set aside. Thoroughly combine all the remaining ingredients in a large bowl. Stir in the sautéed onion.

Preheat the oven to 350 degrees. Lightly grease a 9 × 13-inch baking pan. Pour in the cheese-spinach mixture. Bake until firm, about 40 minutes. Let cool slightly. Cut into squares before serving.

Serves 8.

PER SERVING: 136 CAL.; 17G PROT.; 5G FAT; 8G CARB.; 117MG CHOL.; 400MG SOD.; 2.3G FIBER.

Legume Cookery

You may cook legumes by different methods. Some methods are quicker than others, but all get the job done. Lentils, split peas and mung beans need no soaking.

❖ Traditional method: Rinse the legumes and remove any debris, such as tiny stones. (Usually there is nothing to pick out.) Place the legumes in a large pot with 3 to 4 times their volume of water. Cover and soak for 8 hours or overnight. (In warm weather, soak the legumes in your refrigerator to prevent fermentation.) Bring the water and legumes to a boil, reduce the heat to a gentle simmer and cook until done.

❖ Quick-soak method: Rinse the legumes and remove any debris. Place the legumes in a large pot with 3 to 4 times their volume of water. Bring to a boil, remove from the heat and let stand, covered, for 1 hour. Then cook the legumes.

❖ Pressure-cooker method: Soak the legumes by either the traditional or the quick-soak method. Follow the cooker's manufacturer's instructions, making certain that the vents on the cooker don't get clogged with foam. One way to reduce foam is to fill your cooker no more than ⅓ full with water and beans and to add 1 tablespoon of oil.

❖ Slow-cooker method: After soaking by either the traditional or the quick-soak method, place the legumes with 4 times their volume of water in your slow cooker. Cover and cook for 6 to 8 hours.

Cooking Times

Times vary according to type and age of legumes, the simmering temperature and the soaking time. One way to know the legumes are cooked is by taste: Bite into a single legume and see if it's tender. If it's tough, cook the legumes longer; if it's mushy, you've overcooked them. Never add salt to the soaking or cooking water unless your recipe instructs otherwise; salt makes the legumes tough.

For every cup of dried legumes, you'll end up with 2¼ to 2½ cups of cooked legumes.

Legumes	Presoak	Cooking Time
Adzuki beans	yes	45 to 60 minutes
Black beans	yes	1 to 1½ hours
Black-eyed peas	yes	1 to ¼ hours
Chickpeas	yes	2½ to 3 hours
Great northern beans	yes	1½ to 2 hours
Kidney beans	yes	1½ to 2½ hours
Lentils	no	30 to 45 minutes
Lima beans (small)	yes	45 to 75 minutes
Lima beans (large)	yes	1 to 1½ hours
Mung beans	no	45 to 60 minutes
Navy beans	yes	1 to 2 hours
Pinto beans	yes	1½ to 2½ hours
Red beans	yes	1½ to 2½ hours
Soybeans	yes	3 or more hours
Split peas	no	45 to 60 minutes

Cheesy Potato Pancakes

Served with applesauce and fresh fruit, this main dish satisfies children's hunger.

1 egg or equivalent egg substitute

⅓ cup skim milk

½ teaspoon salt

3 tablespoons unbleached white flour

1 small onion, diced

¼ to ½ cup shredded reduced-fat cheddar cheese

4 potatoes, peeled and grated

1 to 2 teaspoons safflower or canola oil

In a bowl, whisk together the egg or egg substitute, milk, salt and flour. Add the onion, cheese and potatoes. Heat the oil over medium heat in a large skillet. Pour in about 3 tablespoons of batter per pancake. Cook until the bottom is lightly browned, then turn over and cook the other side. Remove from the skillet. Repeat with the remaining batter. Serve warm.

Serves 4.

PER SERVING: 182 CAL.; 6G PROT.; 3G FAT; 34G CARB.; 5MG CHOL.; 334MG SOD.; 3G FIBER.

Savory 'n' Sweet Rice

Bursting with the good nutrition of carrots, raisins and brown rice, this main dish is healthful and delicious.

1 cup uncooked brown rice

1¾ cups water

3 carrots, shredded

2 eggs, lightly beaten, or equivalent egg substitute

½ cup evaporated skim milk

1 teaspoon salt

½ teaspoon freshly ground black pepper

1 small onion, minced

½ to 1 cup shredded reduced-fat cheddar cheese (optional)

½ cup raisins

¾ cup breadcrumbs, preferably whole wheat

2 tablespoons butter or margarine

Place the rice and water in a medium saucepan, cover and bring to a boil over high heat. Reduce the heat and simmer until tender, about 45 minutes. Drain if necessary.

Preheat the oven to 350 degrees. In a large bowl, combine the rice and all the remaining ingredients except the breadcrumbs and butter or margarine. Mix well. Pour the rice mixture into a lightly greased 8 × 8-inch baking pan. In a small bowl, stir together the breadcrumbs and butter or margarine with a fork or your fingertips until thoroughly combined. Sprinkle over the rice mixture. Bake until firm, about 30 to 40 minutes. Let sit 10 minutes before cutting into squares.

Serves 6.

PER SERVING: 222 CAL.; 7G PROT.; 7G FAT; 34G CARB.; 82MG CHOL.; 573MG SOD.; 3G FIBER.

Lean Bean Burritos

1 teaspoon safflower or canola oil

1 clove garlic, chopped

1 tablespoon chili powder

1 16-ounce can red kidney beans or pinto beans, rinsed

6 tortillas, preferably whole wheat, warmed

¼ cup chopped scallions (green and white parts) or onion

1 cup shredded lettuce

½ cup shredded reduced-fat cheddar cheese (optional)

½ cup mild salsa

In a skillet over medium-high heat, heat the oil and cook the garlic until it starts to brown. Stir in the chili powder. Add the beans, mashing them with a fork while stirring. Add water as necessary to achieve desired consistency.

Divide the bean mixture among the 6 tortillas. Sprinkle with scallions or onion, lettuce and cheese if desired. Top each tortilla with about 1 tablespoon of salsa. Roll the tortillas to close. Fasten each with a toothpick if desired.

VARIATIONS:

❖ For QUICK LEAN BEAN BURRITOS, substitute a 16-ounce can of fat-free refried beans for the first 4 ingredients. Spoon about 2 or 3 tablespoons of the refried beans on each tortilla. Roll up and microwave on high for 30 to 45 seconds. Stuff with desired toppings and serve.

❖ For LEAN BEAN TACOS, spoon the bean mixture into taco shells. Place the taco shells on a baking sheet and heat in a 375-degree oven until heated through, about 5 to 10 minutes. Stuff with desired toppings and serve.

Serves 6.

PER SERVING: 168 CAL.; 8G PROT.; 2G FAT; 37G CARB.; 0 CHOL.; 933MG SOD.; 6.1G FIBER.

Casserole Olé

This dish has just a touch of fire. Grown-ups can add a few drops of red hot sauce to their portions if desired.

1 teaspoon safflower or canola oil

1 teaspoon water

1 to 2 teaspoons minced garlic

3 scallions (green and white parts), sliced

1 red or green bell pepper, cored and chopped

1 teaspoon ground cumin

1 tablespoon chili powder

1 cup whole-kernel corn

1 16-ounce can kidney beans, rinsed

1 cup tomato sauce

6 7-inch corn tortillas

1 cup part-skim ricotta cheese

½ cup shredded reduced-fat cheddar cheese

In a medium skillet over medium-high heat, heat the safflower or canola oil and water, and sauté the garlic, scallions and bell pepper until softened, about 5 minutes. Stir in the cumin and chili powder and cook a few minutes more. Add the corn, beans and tomato sauce. Remove from the heat.

Preheat the oven to 350 degrees. In a lightly greased, 2-quart casserole dish, arrange 3 tortillas to cover the bottom. Top with half of the vegetable mixture. Using a teaspoon, dollop half of the ricotta over the vegetable mixture. Sprinkle on half of the cheddar. Repeat the layers, ending with the cheddar. Bake 30 minutes. Let cool slightly before serving.

Serves 4.

PER SERVING: 394 CAL.; 22G PROT.; 11G FAT; 56G CARB.; 29MG CHOL.; 1,166MG SOD.; 10.3G FIBER.

Bean and Spinach Cassoulet

1 cup dried great northern beans, soaked overnight in 3 cups cold water

3 cups fresh water

1 onion, quartered

1 large clove garlic, halved

1 10-ounce package frozen chopped spinach, thawed and squeezed dry

3 carrots, sliced

½ pound white button mushrooms, thickly sliced

8 ounces tomato puree

1 teaspoon dried Italian seasoning

Freshly ground black pepper to taste

½ cup low-fat cottage cheese

½ cup shredded part-skim mozzarella cheese

1 tablespoon grated Parmesan cheese, preferably fresh

Drain the beans and place them in a large pot with the fresh water, onion and garlic. Bring to a boil, reduce the heat, cover and simmer until barely tender, about 40 minutes. Drain again and discard the garlic. In a medium bowl, combine the spinach, carrots, mushrooms, tomato puree, Italian seasoning and black pepper.

Preheat the oven to 375 degrees. To assemble the cassoulet, spread half of the bean mixture in a 2-quart casserole dish. Spoon half of the cottage cheese on top. Top with half of the vegetable mixture. Repeat the layers. Sprinkle the mozzarella and Parmesan on top. Bake, uncovered, for 45 minutes.

Serves 6.

PER SERVING: 192 CAL.; 15G PROT.; 3G FAT; 30G CARB.; 8MG CHOL.; 222MG SOD.; 9G FIBER.

Green Peppers Stuffed with Basmati Rice and Chickpeas

This remake of traditional high-fat stuffed green peppers bursts with flavor and has only 1 gram of fat per serving.

6 green bell peppers

Water

3 cups cooked basmati rice

1 cup cooked chickpeas (see note)

2 carrots, shredded

1 cup whole-kernel corn

½ onion, chopped

½ cup raisins

½ to 1 cup shredded part-skim mozzarella cheese (optional)

3 to 4 cups tomato sauce

Salt and freshly ground black pepper to taste

Cut the tops from the green peppers. Discard the seeds and membranes. Chop enough of the tops to make ¼ cup. Set aside. Fill a large pot about ⅔ full with the water; bring to a boil and cook the whole green peppers for 5 minutes. Remove and invert to dry.

In a large bowl, combine the remaining ingredients and reserved chopped green pepper.

Preheat the oven to 350 degrees. Cut the peppers in half lengthwise and stuff each half with the rice-bean mixture. Place them in a 9 × 13-inch baking pan. Bake 30 minutes. Transfer the peppers to a platter. Serve warm.

NOTE: Garbanzo bean is another name for chickpea.

Serves 6.

PER SERVING: 278 CAL.; 8G PROT.;
1G FAT; 59G CARB.; 1MG CHOL.;
654MG SOD.; 7G FIBER.

Savory Baked Samosas

A North Indian wrapped food, samosas are customarily fried. Not so in this delicious version.

4 to 5 large potatoes, peeled and diced

1 cup frozen peas

2 tablespoons peanut oil

1 to 2 onions, diced

Up to 1-inch piece fresh gingerroot, peeled and minced

2 cloves garlic, minced

2 teaspoons curry powder

2 teaspoons ground coriander

⅛ teaspoon ground turmeric (optional)

⅛ teaspoon ground cumin (optional)

Salt to taste

1 17¼-ounce package thawed puff pastry shells

About ¼ cup unbleached white flour, for dusting

In a large pot, boil the potatoes until very tender. Drain. Place the peas in a colander and let thaw under running water. Transfer the potatoes and peas to a large bowl.

In a large skillet over medium heat, heat the oil. Add the onions, ginger and garlic and cook until the onions are transparent, about 10 minutes. Add the curry powder, coriander, and turmeric and cumin if desired. Raise the heat and cook 5 minutes more. Add the onion mixture to the bowl and mash the mixture coarsely. Season with the salt. Set aside.

To prepare the pastry, cut each piece of dough into 3 equal panels, then cut each panel into 2¼-inch squares; you will have 18 squares. Dust your work surface with the flour. Roll out the dough pieces to twice their size. If necessary, use your fingers to spread the dough into shape. Place 1 heaping tablespoon of the vegetable mixture in the center of each square and fold over 1 corner to make a triangle. Pinch the sides to enclose the mixture.

Preheat the oven to 350 degrees. Place the samosas 1 inch apart on baking sheets. Bake until golden, about 25 minutes. Serve hot.

Makes 18 samosas.

PER SAMOSA: 276 CAL.; 5G PROT.; 16G FAT; 28G CARB.; 5MG CHOL.; 211MG SOD.; 2.4G FIBER.

Apricot and Bulgur Stuffed Crepes

This savory dish tastes absolutely wonderful as is or topped with Brown Gravy (page 198).

CREPES

  1 egg

  ¾ cup skim milk

Dash salt

  ½ cup unbleached white flour

STUFFING

  2 teaspoons butter or margarine

  1 onion, chopped

  ½ cup chopped white button mushrooms

  ½ cup uncooked bulgur

  1 cup water

  ⅓ cup dried apricots, chopped

  2 tablespoons chopped toasted pecans

Salt to taste

Crepes: Combine the crepe ingredients in a blender or food processor and whirl until smooth. Pour into a small bowl. Let sit 30 minutes.

Stuffing: In a medium saucepan over medium heat, heat the butter or margarine and sauté the onion and mushrooms until the onion is transparent, about 10 minutes. Add the bulgur and water. Bring to a boil, cover and simmer 20 to 30 minutes. Stir in the apricots, pecans and salt. Set aside.

To make the crepes, lightly coat an 8-inch nonstick skillet with vegetable oil cooking spray. Heat the skillet over medium heat. Using 2 to 3 tablespoons of batter per crepe, pour the batter into the center of the skillet, gently tilting it so the batter spreads to the edges. Cook 30 to 40 seconds. Loosen an edge of the crepe with a spatula and flip over. Cook 15 seconds more. Slide the crepe onto a sheet of waxed paper. Repeat this process until all the batter is used up, stacking the crepes between sheets of waxed paper.

Place a crepe on a plate. Spread about 3 tablespoons of the stuffing over half of the crepe and fold the crepe over. Transfer to a 9 × 13-inch baking pan. Repeat this process with the remaining crepes and stuffing. Serve warm.

For APRICOT AND BULGUR PILAF, omit the crepes and double the stuffing ingredients. Proceed with the recipe as directed.

Makes 8; serves 4.

PER SERVING: 225 CAL.; 8G PROT.; 6G FAT; 37G CARB.; 47MG CHOL.; 263MG SOD.; 5.6G FIBER.

Vegetable Curry with Basmati Rice

Packed with vegetables, this curry has lots of vitamins and minerals as well as South Indian flair. You may substitute any other vegetables for the ones listed here. Try sweet potatoes, broccoli, eggplant or green plantain.

2 carrots, cut into ¼-inch rounds

1 cup cauliflower florets

2 red potatoes, peeled and cubed

½ cup green beans

1 4-ounce can minced green chilies

About ¾ cup water

1 teaspoon fresh lemon juice or lime juice

3 tablespoons grated unsweetened coconut

1 to 2 teaspoons curry powder

½ cup nonfat plain yogurt, at room temperature

Salt to taste

1¾ cups water

1 cup uncooked basmati rice

In a medium saucepan, combine the carrots, cauliflower, potatoes, green beans, chilies and about ¾ cup water. Cover and cook over medium heat until the vegetables are tender but not mushy, about 15 minutes. Add the lemon or lime juice, coconut and curry powder. Gradually stir the yogurt into the vegetable mixture. Season with the salt.

In another saucepan, bring the 1 ¾ cups water to a boil. Add the rice, cover and simmer until the liquid is absorbed, about 15 minutes. Serve the curry over the rice.

Serves 6.

PER SERVING: 154 CAL.; 4G PROT.; 2G FAT; 31G CARB.; 4MG CHOL.; 34MG SOD.; 2.8G FIBER.

Black Bean Chili

This thick chili tastes great with hunks of corn bread. Add extra chili powder and cayenne pepper to the chili for a spicier flavor.

3 cups cooked black beans

½ to 1 cup cooked brown rice

½ to 1 onion, chopped

1 red bell pepper, cored and chopped

2 cloves garlic, minced

1 28-ounce can tomatoes, chopped, with juice

1 tablespoon chili powder

1 teaspoon ground cumin

Dash cayenne pepper

Salt and freshly ground black pepper to taste

¾ cup whole-kernel corn

In a large pot, combine all the ingredients except the corn and heat on medium-high until simmering. Reduce the heat and let simmer for 1 hour. Add the corn during the last 10 minutes of cooking. Serve warm.

Serves 6.

PER SERVING: 188 CAL.; 10G PROT.; 1G FAT; 37G CARB.; 0 CHOL.; 104MG SOD.; 12.5G FIBER.

Skinny Shepherd's Pie

This delicious and colorful version of shepherd's pie has 3 grams of fat in a hefty serving.

1 to 2 teaspoons minced garlic

1 large onion, sliced

1 cup green beans

2 carrots, sliced

3 baking potatoes, peeled and cut into chunks

1 sweet potato, peeled and cut into chunks

½ pound sliced white button mushrooms

2 cups water

2 tablespoons soy sauce or tamari

¼ cup apple juice

½ teaspoon dried oregano

½ teaspoon dried thyme

Freshly ground black pepper to taste

3 to 4 tablespoons arrowroot or cornstarch dissolved in ¼ cup water

2 to 3 cups Sour Cream Whipped Potatoes (see recipe, page 191) or your favorite mashed potatoes

In a large pot, combine all the ingredients except the dissolved arrowroot or cornstarch and whipped potatoes. Bring to a boil, cover and reduce the heat. Simmer until the vegetables are tender, about 40 minutes. Slowly add the dissolved arrowroot or cornstarch to the pot, stirring constantly until thickened.

Preheat the oven to 350 degrees. Spoon into a lightly greased 9 × 13-inch baking pan. Dollop the whipped potatoes on top. Bake until the potatoes are lightly browned, about 25 to 30 minutes. Serve warm.

VARIATION:

For HEARTY VEGETABLE STEW, omit the whipped potatoes and spoon the stew straight from the pot into individual bowls.

Serves 8.

PER SERVING: 569 CAL.; 5G PROT.; 3G FAT; 133G CARB.; 0 CHOL.; 365MG SOD.; 5.8G FIBER.

Pineapple-Peanut Bow Ties

Reminiscent of Thai cuisine, this noodle dish plays up a kid-friendly favorite: peanut butter.

12 ounces uncooked bow ties or other pasta shape

¼ cup peanut butter

¼ cup skim milk or reduced-fat soy milk

¼ cup crushed pineapple, drained

1 scallion (green and white parts), sliced

Dash cayenne pepper

Chopped peanuts for garnish

Cook the pasta according to package directions. In a small saucepan over medium-low heat, warm the peanut butter and milk, stirring constantly, until smooth. Remove from the heat. Stir in the pineapple, scallion and cayenne. Combine with the cooked pasta. Garnish with the chopped peanuts.

Serves 4.

PER SERVING: 442 CAL.; 16G PROT.; 10G FAT; 74G CARB.; 1MG CHOL.; 16MG SOD.; 4G FIBER.

Sunburst Burgers

Dress up these burgers with your favorite trimmings: lettuce, tomato slices, pickle slices, mustard and ketchup.

2¼ cups water

2 to 3 tablespoons soy sauce or tamari

1 onion, minced

3 tablespoons sunflower seeds

1 clove garlic, minced

1 teaspoon dried Italian seasoning or dried oregano

2 cups rolled oats

8 whole-wheat burger buns

Combine all the ingredients except the rolled oats and buns in a medium pot. Bring to a boil. Stir in the rolled oats, reduce the heat and cook for 5 minutes, stirring frequently. Let cool.

Preheat the oven to 350 degrees. Lightly oil a large baking sheet. Wet your hands and shape the oat mixture into 8 patties. Bake 20 minutes on the first side and 10 to 15 minutes on the second. Serve on the buns.

HELPFUL HINT: These patties freeze well, so make extra burgers for quick dinners and lunches. Simply double the ingredients and prepare as directed. Place extra patties in an airtight container and freeze. To warm through, let the burgers thaw, then place under a broiler for a few minutes.

Makes 8 burgers.
PER BURGER: 214 CAL.; 9G PROT.; 5G FAT; 35G CARB.; 0 CHOL.; 481MG SOD.; 4G FIBER.

Natural Peanut Butter vs. the Brand Names

Natural peanut butter has no additives, so it tastes less sweet and salty than brand-name peanut butter. It also separates as the oil naturally rises to the surface. To make it smooth, simply stir together the contents of the peanut butter jar before using. The brand names usually have added stabilizers, usually hydrogenated oil, to prevent separation. Check labels.

So is natural better? If you want to avoid additives, yes. If you value convenience, no. Not only does natural peanut butter need to be stirred, it also must be refrigerated to prevent rancidity. But natural peanut butter has a bonus for weight watchers: Some of the oil may be poured off to reduce fat content. Expect this slimmed-down peanut butter to stick to the roof of your mouth unless you add a little water, apple juice or nonfat plain yogurt to a portion before eating it.

Interestingly, peanut butter manufacturers, which have spiked their products with salt and sugar for years, are now touting low-sugar, low-salt and reduced-fat versions. Read product labels before making your purchase.

Sloppy Joeys

Textured vegetable protein, or TVP (a registered trademark of the Archer-Daniels-Midland Company), makes a great replacement for ground beef in this childhood favorite.

⅞ cup boiling water

1 cup textured vegetable protein granules

2 teaspoons virgin olive oil

½ onion, chopped

1 clove garlic, minced

½ cup minced green bell pepper

3 ounces tomato paste

⅓ to ½ cup ketchup

1 teaspoon dried Italian seasoning or dried oregano

2 teaspoons vegetarian Worcestershire sauce

1 to 2 teaspoons honey or sugar (optional)

About ½ cup water

Dash cayenne pepper

Salt and freshly ground black pepper to taste

4 whole-wheat burger buns

In a small bowl, pour the boiling water over the textured vegetable protein granules. Let sit until the water is absorbed, about 10 minutes. Meanwhile, in a saucepan over medium heat, heat the olive oil and sauté the onion, garlic and green pepper until the onion is transparent, about 10 minutes. Add the textured vegetable protein granules and continue cooking another 5 minutes.

In a medium bowl, combine the tomato paste, ketchup, Italian seasoning or oregano, Worcestershire sauce, honey or sugar if desired and enough water to make a thick sauce. Pour the sauce into the saucepan and stir until combined. Season with the cayenne, salt and black pepper. Add a bit more water as necessary. Cook 5 to 10 minutes more. Spoon over the bottom half of the burger buns, cover with the tops and serve warm.

VARIATION:

For BARBECUED SLOPPY JOEYS, replace the ketchup with your favorite barbecue sauce.

Serves 4.

PER SERVING: 264 CAL.; 15G PROT.; 5G FAT; 41G CARB.; 0 CHOL.; 583MG SOD.; 5G FIBER.

Great Bean Lunch Spread

This spread is versatile: You can use it on bread for sandwiches, spoon it into pita rounds and add shredded carrots, tomato slices and lettuce for a light meal, or serve it on crackers for a snack or as part of a finger-food meal.

½ cup fresh parsley, chopped

1 16-ounce can great northern beans, rinsed

2 tablespoons fresh lemon juice

Dash salt

2 to 4 tablespoons nonfat plain yogurt (optional)

In a medium bowl, combine all the ingredients, mashing the beans with a fork until a few lumps remain. Stir well. Chill.

VARIATION:

Substitute pinto beans or red kidney beans for the great northern beans.

Makes 10 2-tablespoon servings.
PER SERVING: 54 CAL.; 3G PROT.; 0.2G FAT; 10G CARB.; 0 CHOL.; 30MG SOD.; 2.3G FIBER.

Super Simple Sandwich Spread

The ingredients list may appear too simple to make great-tasting sandwiches, but don't be fooled. It's delicious. If you wish, jazz up the sandwiches by adding your favorite fixings, such as lettuce, tomatoes, pickles and shredded carrots.

1 16-ounce can red beans, rinsed

2 scallions (light green and white parts), chopped

In a medium bowl, mash together the beans and scallions with the back of a spoon until almost smooth. Chill.

Makes 8 2-tablespoon servings.
PER SERVING: 69 CAL.; 5G PROT.; 0.5G FAT; 13G CARB.; 0 CHOL.; 2MG SOD.; 3.5G FIBER.

Low-Fat PB&J

The peanut butter and jelly sandwich is a kid's favorite. In this version, the peanut butter is cut with reduced-fat tofu or part-skim ricotta cheese, lowering fat content and adding calcium.

2 tablespoons peanut butter

2 tablespoons reduced-fat tofu or part-skim ricotta cheese

About 3 tablespoons jelly or fruit spread

8 slices whole-wheat bread

In a small bowl, using a fork, thoroughly combine the peanut butter and tofu or ricotta. Spread about 1 tablespoon of the peanut butter mixture on a slice of bread and about 2 teaspoons of jelly or fruit spread on another slice of bread to make a sandwich. Repeat to make 4 sandwiches. Refrigerate any leftover peanut butter spread.

VARIATION:

In place of jelly or fruit spread, use banana slices, apple slices or raisins.

Makes 4 sandwiches.

PER SANDWICH: 226 CAL.; 8G PROT.; 5G FAT; 37G CARB.; 0 CHOL.; 345MG SOD.; 4.6G FIBER.

Fruit 'n' Cream Cheese Bagel

4 tablespoons low-fat cream cheese

2 raisin bagels, cut in half and lightly toasted

Ground cinnamon to taste

1 banana, sliced

1 kiwi, peeled and sliced

Spread 1 tablespoon cream cheese on each bagel half. Sprinkle with the cinnamon. Layer the banana and kiwi on top. Serve.

VARIATION:

Use peach slices in place of the banana or kiwi.

Serves 4.

PER SERVING: 163 CAL.; 5G PROT.; 4G FAT; 30G CARB.; 5MG CHOL.; 236MG SOD.; 2.4G FIBER.

Sour Cream Whipped Potatoes

Butter and milk weigh down traditional mashed potatoes. This version calls on nonfat sour cream, a bit of reduced-fat margarine and a few dashes of salt to make a healthful side dish.

8 potatoes, peeled and cut into chunks

Water to cover

2 tablespoons nonfat sour cream

2 tablespoons reduced-fat margarine or butter

¼ teaspoon salt, or to taste

In a large pot, bring the potatoes and water to a boil. Cook until fork-tender, about 20 minutes. Drain well. Add the sour cream and margarine or butter to the pot. Whip with an electric beater until smooth. Add the salt and whip again. Serve warm.

Serves 8.

PER SERVING: 137 CAL.; 3G PROT.; 2G FAT; 28G CARB.; 0 CHOL.; 62MG SOD.; 2.4G FIBER.

Breakfast Your Way

OH-MY OATMEAL: Cook rolled oats according to package directions. Stir in any of the following, alone or in combination: raisins, ground cinnamon, shredded coconut, sliced bananas, maple syrup, chopped dried apricots, brown sugar.

BETTER PANCAKES: Replace ¼ to ½ the amount of white flour in your favorite pancake recipe with whole-wheat flour. Top the pancakes with a warm fruit topping, such as blueberries, raspberries or sliced apples.

BREAKFAST BURRITO: Lightly sauté chopped green and red bell peppers, chopped onion and thinly sliced potatoes, adding 1 or 2 scrambled eggs if desired. Then stuff the mixture into burritos.

TOAST EXTRAVAGANZA: After toasting your favorite bread, top the slices with a smear of honey and sliced fruit; some cream cheese or cottage cheese and a sprinkle of ground cinnamon; or a fruity chutney.

Polenta with Chunky Tomato Sauce

3 cups water, divided

Pinch salt

1 cup cornmeal

1 cup Chunky Tomato Sauce (see recipe, page 197) or your favorite store-bought tomato sauce

¼ cup grated Parmesan cheese, preferably fresh (optional)

To make the polenta, bring 2 cups water to a boil in a medium pot. Add the salt. Slowly stir in the cornmeal, then reduce the heat to medium. Slowly stir in the remaining 1 cup water. Cook for about 5 minutes while stirring constantly. Remove from the heat.

Preheat the oven to 350 degrees. Coat the bottom of a 9 × 13-inch baking pan with a ladle of sauce. Using a large spoon, place half of the polenta in the pan, 1 spoonful at a time. Cover the polenta with half of the sauce. Sprinkle with half of the Parmesan if desired. Repeat the layers, ending with the Parmesan. Bake until heated through, about 25 minutes. Serve warm.

Serves 8.

PER SERVING: 77 CAL.; 2G PROT.; 0.3G FAT; 16G CARB.; 0 CHOL.; 116MG SOD.; 1.8G FIBER.

Baked Potatoes with Toppings

Potatoes may be topped in so many delicious ways. Here are some ideas.

4 large potatoes, scrubbed

1 to 2 teaspoons safflower or canola oil

Toppings: salsa and black beans; thick tomato sauce and shredded part-skim mozzarella cheese; sautéed shiitake mushrooms; sauerkraut, diced red apple and caraway seeds; sliced scallions, pitted Greek olives and crumbled feta cheese; mixed steamed vegetables

2 to 4 tablespoons nonfat plain yogurt (optional)

Preheat the oven to 400 degrees. Rub the potato skins lightly with the safflower or canola oil. Place the potatoes on a baking sheet and bake until tender, about 45 minutes.

Make a slit in each potato. Using your fingers, press the potatoes to loosen the pulp. Spoon in a topping of your choice. Dollop the yogurt on top if desired. Serve warm.

Serves 4.

PER SERVING: 155 CAL.; 3G PROT.; 1G FAT; 34G CARB.; 0 CHOL.; 8MG SOD.; 2.3G FIBER.

Spanish Rice

Here's a flavorful accompaniment to any Spanish-themed dish. Add cayenne pepper when you want to turn up the heat.

- 2 teaspoons safflower or canola oil
- ½ onion, chopped
- ½ cup diced green bell pepper
- ½ cup chopped white button mushrooms
- 1 4-ounce can minced green chilies (see note)
- 2 cups cooked brown rice
- 1 to 1½ cups tomato sauce
- ½ teaspoon dried basil
- ½ teaspoon dried oregano
- ½ teaspoon chili powder
- Salt to taste

In a saucepan over medium heat, heat the safflower or canola oil and sauté the onion, green pepper and mushrooms until the onion is transparent, about 10 minutes. Stir in the remaining ingredients and cook, stirring occasionally, for 20 minutes. Serve warm.

NOTE: Use only 1 tablespoon of green chilies if you want a mild dish.

VARIATION:

To turn this dish into an entrée, add 1 cup of cooked legumes of your choice. Red kidney beans and black beans are good choices.

Serves 4.

PER SERVING: 170 CAL.; 4G PROT.; 3G FAT; 32G CARB.; 0 CHOL.; 444MG SOD.; 4G FIBER.

Cool Cucumber Raita

Raita is a traditional Indian side dish that provides a refreshing contrast to curries. It works well with any main dish in which you want a cooling complement.

2 cups nonfat plain yogurt

1 to 2 teaspoons ground cumin

1 tablespoon fresh lemon juice

Salt to taste

2 cucumbers, seeded and thinly sliced

2 tablespoons minced fresh parsley

In a serving dish, whisk together the yogurt, cumin, lemon juice and salt. Stir in the cucumbers and parsley. Chill.

Serves 4.

PER SERVING: 93 CAL.; 8G PROT.; 1G FAT; 14G CARB.; 2MG CHOL.; 234MG SOD.; 1G FIBER.

Three-Fruit Kebabs

Here's an eye-appealing way to serve fruit as breakfast or as a side dish at dinner. Be sure to blunt the ends of your skewers.

2 red apples, cored and cut into 6 slices per apple

2 cups seedless green grapes (see note)

2 oranges, white pith removed, sectioned

6 wooden skewers

Thread the fruits, alternating them, onto the skewers. Place them attractively on a platter.

NOTE: When serving these kebabs to young children, be sure to cut the grapes in half.

VARIATION:

Substitute 1 cup pineapple chunks, 3 kiwis (peeled and thickly sliced) and 1 pint strawberries (stems removed) for the apples, grapes and oranges.

Serves 6.

PER SERVING: 68 CAL.; 1G PROT.; 0.3G FAT; 18G CARB.; 0 CHOL.; 1MG SOD.; 2.7G FIBER.

Raspberry Applesauce

6 Rome Beauty or other sweet apples, peeled, cored and chopped

½ cup apple juice

⅔ cup frozen unsweetened raspberries (see note)

In a medium saucepan, cook the apples with the apple juice until tender, about 30 minutes. Mash with a fork to achieve a chunky consistency. Add the raspberries, stirring gently, until heated through, about 10 minutes. Serve warm.

NOTE: If you can't find the unsweetened type, use sweetened raspberries and rinse them before adding to the applesauce.

Serves 6.

PER SERVING: 96 CAL.; 1G PROT.; 1G FAT; 25G CARB.; 0 CHOL.; 1MG SOD.; 3.8G FIBER.

Vegetable Stock

You may use this as a broth or as an ingredient in recipes. Choose unpeeled, washed vegetables. You may vary the flavor by adding your favorite herbs or other vegetables. Just stay away from strongly flavored vegetables like asparagus, broccoli, cabbage and cauliflower. You may freeze the stock in small quantities by using ice cube trays for freezing; once frozen, place the cubes in large zipper-type bags and store in the freezer. Then remove them as needed.

2 onions, quartered

3 carrots, thickly sliced

2 celery stalks with greens, thickly sliced

½ bunch fresh parsley

3 potatoes, quartered

2 tomatoes, quartered

4 cloves garlic

8 peppercorns

1 bay leaf

8 cups water

In a large saucepan, combine all the ingredients and bring to boiling over high heat. Reduce the heat, cover and simmer for 1 hour. Strain the stock and discard the vegetables, garlic, peppercorns and bay leaf. Let cool. Refrigerate.

Makes 8 cups.

PER CUP: 54 CAL.; 2G PROT.; 0 FAT; 12G CARB.; 0 CHOL.; 20MG SOD.; 0 FIBER.

Chunky Tomato Sauce

½ cup red wine

1 teaspoon minced garlic

½ onion, cut into wedges

1 carrot, minced

4 white button mushrooms, coarsely chopped

1 28-ounce can diced tomatoes

1 6-ounce can tomato paste

1 teaspoon dried oregano

Freshly ground black pepper to taste

1 bay leaf

Salt to taste

Dash nutmeg

In a medium saucepan over medium-high heat, bring the wine to a boil and sauté the garlic, onion, carrot and mushrooms until the liquid evaporates. Add the tomatoes and cook 15 minutes more. Stir in the tomato paste, oregano and pepper. Add the bay leaf. Reduce the heat and simmer, uncovered, for 30 to 60 minutes. Stir in the salt and nutmeg. Remove the bay leaf. Serve.

VARIATION:

For a smoother sauce, finely chop the onion and mushrooms before sautéing.

Makes 3 cups.

PER ½ CUP: 106 CAL.; 4G PROT.; 0.3G FAT; 21G CARB.; 0 CHOL.; 808MG SOD.; 3.3G FIBER.

Brown Gravy

2 teaspoons safflower or
canola oil

½ onion, diced

½ teaspoon minced garlic

½ cup whole-wheat flour

2 cups vegetable stock or
water

2 to 4 tablespoons low-
sodium soy sauce or
tamari

Freshly ground black pepper
to taste

In a saucepan over medium heat, heat the safflower or canola oil and sauté the onion and garlic until the onion is transparent, about 7 minutes. Blend in the flour and cook until lightly toasted, about 2 minutes. Reduce the heat. Slowly add the vegetable stock or water and soy sauce or tamari, and cook, stirring often, until thickened, about 5 minutes. Add more water as necessary to achieve desired consistency. Transfer to a serving dish and serve warm.

VARIATION:

For MUSHROOM GRAVY, sauté 1 cup sliced white button mushrooms in 1 teaspoon safflower oil until the mushrooms begin to exude moisture. Stir the sautéed mushrooms and their juice into the warm gravy.

Makes about 2 cups.

PER 2 TABLESPOONS: 21 CAL.; 1G PROT.; 1G FAT; 3G CARB.; 0 CHOL.; 75MG SOD.; 0.5G FIBER.

12

Ends

These desserts are both nutritious and delicious. Because they have redeeming nutritional profiles—with most of them scoring low in fat—make them a part of your meals. When you're not in the mood to fix dessert, place a platter of sliced fruit on the table and delight in nature's sweetness.

Chocolate Brownie Cake

A cross between a brownie and a cake, this richly flavored but relatively low-fat dessert is perfect to serve at a birthday or anytime you desire a healthful indulgence. Surprisingly, it contains neither eggs nor dairy products.

CAKE

½ cup whole-wheat flour or unbleached white flour

2 cups unbleached white flour

1½ cups sugar

½ cup unsweetened cocoa powder

2 teaspoons baking soda

½ teaspoon salt

2 cups water

6 tablespoons safflower or canola oil

2 tablespoons white distilled vinegar

1 teaspoon vanilla extract

GLAZE

1 cup confectioners' sugar

3 to 4 tablespoons unsweetened cocoa powder

2 to 3 tablespoons reduced-fat soy milk or skim milk

Cake: Preheat the oven to 350 degrees. Lightly grease and flour 2 8-inch cake pans. In a large bowl, combine the dry ingredients. In a separate bowl, mix together the remaining ingredients and pour them into the dry ingredients, stirring until just combined. Pour the batter into the prepared pans. Bake until a toothpick inserted in the center comes out clean, about 35 minutes. Let cool 10 minutes in the pans, then transfer to wire racks.

Glaze: Mix together the confectioners' sugar and cocoa powder in a small bowl. Stir in the soy milk or skim milk 1 tablespoon at a time until the glaze reaches a thick, pouring consistency.

Place 1 cake layer on a cake stand or platter. Coat with the glaze, then top with the second cake layer. Spread the glaze over the sides and top of the cake.

VARIATION:

If you don't mind the extra calories and fat, use chocolate frosting in place of the glaze.

Serves 8.

PER SERVING: 433 CAL.; 5G PROT.; 12G FAT; 82G CARB.; 0 CHOL.; 451MG SOD.; 4.1G FIBER.

Apple Streusel Cake

½ cup whole-wheat pastry flour, whole-wheat flour or unbleached white flour

1 cup unbleached white flour

⅔ cup sugar

2 teaspoons baking powder

½ teaspoon salt

1 egg, lightly beaten, or equivalent egg substitute

½ cup skim milk

2½ tablespoons safflower or canola oil

½ small banana, mashed

½ cup raisins

2 apples, cored, peeled and thinly sliced

¼ cup packed brown sugar

1 tablespoon unbleached white flour

1 tablespoon margarine or butter, softened

1½ teaspoons ground cinnamon

In a medium bowl, combine the flours, sugar, baking powder and salt. In a large bowl, whisk together the egg or egg substitute, skim milk, safflower or canola oil and banana. Add the flour mixture, stirring until just combined. Fold in the raisins.

Preheat the oven to 375 degrees. Lightly grease an 8 × 8-inch baking pan. Spoon in half of the batter. Top with the apple slices and the remaining batter.

In a small bowl, combine the remaining ingredients, using a fork or your fingers, until the mixture resembles crumbs. Sprinkle over the batter. Bake 25 to 30 minutes.

Makes 9 squares.

PER SQUARE: 243 CAL.; 4G PROT.; 6G FAT; 46G CARB.; 24MG CHOL.; 253MG SOD.; 2.6G FIBER.

Banana-ana Bread

Loaded with bananas and light on fat, this dessert is a healthful treat. In fact, it can make a great start to the day.

½ cup whole-wheat pastry flour, whole-wheat flour or unbleached white flour

¾ cup unbleached white flour

½ cup sugar

¾ teaspoon baking powder

½ teaspoon baking soda

Scant ½ teaspoon salt

3 tablespoons reduced-fat margarine or butter

½ cup plus 2 tablespoons mashed banana

⅓ cup buttermilk, sour milk (see note) or reduced-fat soy milk

2 eggs, lightly beaten, or equivalent egg substitute

½ teaspoon vanilla extract

Preheat the oven to 350 degrees. Lightly grease and flour an 8 × 8-inch baking pan. In a mixing bowl, combine the first 6 ingredients. Add the margarine or butter and banana. Mix with an electric beater on low speed until combined. Add the remaining ingredients and mix on high speed for 2 minutes. Pour the batter into the prepared pan. Bake until a toothpick inserted in the center comes out clean, about 25 to 30 minutes. Let cool. Cut into squares.

NOTE: To make sour milk, pour 1 tablespoon white distilled vinegar into a measuring cup and add milk to measure ⅓ cup.

VARIATION:

To make a delicious banana cake, double the ingredients and pour the batter into 2 greased and floured cake pans. Frost with your favorite cream cheese frosting or dribble a chocolate glaze on top.

Makes 9 squares.

PER SQUARE: 155 CAL.; 4G PROT.; 4G FAT; 27G CARB.; 48MG CHOL.; 276MG SOD.; 1.3G FIBER.

Why White Sugar?

In these recipes, I've called for white sugar—and not the supposedly more healthful sugars like honey, granulated sugarcane juice,
turbinado sugar, barley malt syrup, rice syrup, maple syrup and so
on.

The truth is, sugar is sugar. Except for blackstrap molasses,
which contains a significant amount of iron, and fructose, a highly
refined sugar that can have some health advantages for diabetics,
every other type of sugar lacks redeeming qualities. The amounts
of vitamins and minerals that they might contain are so minute
that they provide no real nutritional advantage.

That's the main reason I opt for white and brown sugar. Brown
sugar, by the way, is just white sugar with a little molasses added
to it. These sugars are easy to use, inexpensive and widely available.
But because sugar is nothing but empty calories, I've kept the
amounts to a minimum.

You, too, can lower your sugar intake by cutting sugar in your
favorite recipes by a third and sometimes a half without losing taste.
In fact, I've found that the flavor of many baked goods and other
dishes *improves* when the sugar is reduced.

In addition, do your body an extra favor by saying no to packaged foods, which often have added sugar. Though sugar isn't the
monster some people believe it is—it does cause tooth decay but
isn't implicated in serious disease, most research shows—the sweet
stuff ought not be overeaten. It's a waste of calories.

Carrot Mini-Muffins

This low-fat dessert also makes a wonderful breakfast. The muffins are rich in beta-carotene, iron and fiber.

1 cup crushed bran flakes cereal

1½ cups whole-wheat flour

¼ cup packed brown sugar

2 teaspoons baking powder

½ teaspoon baking soda

1¼ teaspoons ground cinnamon

¾ teaspoon ground nutmeg

1¼ cups skim milk or reduced-fat soy milk

1 egg or equivalent egg substitute

3 tablespoons safflower or canola oil

1½ cups grated carrots

½ cup raisins

Preheat the oven to 400 degrees. Combine the dry ingredients in a large bowl. Mix together the milk, egg or egg substitute, and safflower or canola oil. Stir the wet ingredients into the dry ingredients until just combined. Fold in the carrots and raisins. Spoon the batter into lightly greased mini-muffin pans or into a 12-cup regular-size muffin pan. Bake until a toothpick inserted in the center comes out clean, about 10 to 15 minutes for mini-muffins and 15 to 20 minutes for regular-size muffins.

Makes about 36 mini-muffins.

PER MINI-MUFFIN: 48 CAL.; 1G PROT.; 1G FAT; 8G CARB.; 6MG CHOL.; 63MG SOD.; 1.1G FIBER.

Cinnamon-Raisin Bread Pudding

4 cups cubed whole-wheat bread

½ cup raisins

1 to 2 teaspoons ground cinnamon

2 12-ounce cans evaporated skim milk

1 egg, lightly beaten, or equivalent egg substitute

¼ cup packed brown sugar

1 teaspoon butter

Place the bread cubes in a greased 8 × 8-inch baking pan. Sprinkle evenly with the raisins and cinnamon. In a small bowl, mix together the evaporated skim milk, egg or egg substitute, and brown sugar. Pour into the pan. With a fork, push down the bread cubes so that they become saturated with the liquid. Let stand for 30 minutes. Dot with butter.

Preheat the oven to 350 degrees. Bake the bread pudding until set, about 1 hour. Let stand 10 minutes before cutting into squares. Serve warm.

Serves 9.

PER SERVING: 165 CAL.; 9G PROT.; 2G FAT; 29G CARB.; 28MG CHOL.; 211MG SOD.; 1.8G FIBER.

Ambrosia

Ambrosia means "the food of the gods." And it is certainly fit for your little ones.

1 orange, white pith removed

1 cup seedless green or red grapes, halved

½ cantaloupe, cut into bite-size pieces

1 cup berries of any kind

4 tablespoons shredded coconut

Cut the orange into bite-size pieces. Layer the orange pieces, grapes, cantaloupe and berries in 4 small bowls or glasses. Sprinkle 1 tablespoon coconut over each portion. Chill.

Serves 4.

PER SERVING: 89 CAL.; 1G PROT.; 2G FAT; 19G CARB.; 0 CHOL.; 19 MG SOD.; 2.8G FIBER.

Oatmeal Chocolate Chip Cookies

4 tablespoons reduced-fat margarine

½ small banana

½ cup packed brown sugar

⅓ cup sugar

1 egg, lightly beaten, or equivalent egg substitute

½ teaspoon vanilla extract

½ cup unbleached white flour

¼ cup whole-wheat flour

½ teaspoon baking soda

½ teaspoon salt

1½ cups rolled oats

1 cup semisweet chocolate chips

Preheat the oven to 375 degrees. In a medium bowl, combine the margarine, banana and sugars with a fork, mashing the mixture to remove any lumps. Whisk in the egg or egg substitute and vanilla. In a small bowl, combine the flours, baking soda and salt. Stir the dry ingredients into the wet ingredients. Add the oats and chocolate chips and combine thoroughly.

Drop the batter by rounded teaspoonfuls onto cookie sheets. Bake until lightly browned, about 10 minutes. Remove from the cookie sheets and place on paper towels to cool. Store in an airtight container.

VARIATION:

For OATMEAL-RAISIN COOKIES, replace the chocolate chips with ¾ cup raisins and add 1 teaspoon ground cinnamon to the dry ingredients before combining with the wet ingredients.

Makes 36 cookies.

PER COOKIE: 78 CAL.; 1G PROT.; 3G FAT; 12G CARB.; 7MG CHOL.; 60MG SOD.; 0.7G FIBER.

Cookie-Cutter Cookies

These not-too-sweet, low-fat treats may be fashioned into pumpkins, Christmas trees, stars, teddy bears or whatever the shape of your cookie cutters. For a festive touch, decorate the cookies with icing and a sprinkle of sugar.

2 cups unbleached white flour

½ teaspoon baking powder

6 tablespoons reduced-fat margarine

¼ cup low-fat cream cheese

⅔ cup sugar

1 egg, lightly beaten, or equivalent egg substitute

½ teaspoon vanilla extract

In a medium bowl, stir together the flour and baking powder. In a separate bowl, beat the margarine and cream cheese until fluffy. Add the remaining ingredients and beat again. Pour in the flour mixture, beating until well blended. Cover and chill for 2 to 3 hours or overnight.

Preheat the oven to 375 degrees. Lightly grease your work surface. Using ¼ of the dough at a time, roll it out to a ⅛-inch thickness. (Keep the remainder of the dough in the refrigerator.) Cut into desired shapes and place on cookie sheets. Bake until lightly browned on the bottom, about 8 to 10 minutes. Remove from the cookie sheets and let cool on paper towels. Decorate the cookies as desired. Store in an airtight container.

Makes 18 large or 36 small cookies.

PER LARGE COOKIE: 110 CAL.; 2G PROT.; 4G FAT; 17G CARB.; 13MG CHOL.; 58MG SOD.; 0.4G FIBER.

Silly Spider Cookies

Invented by my daughter, Laura, these no-bake cookies are fun for kids to make and eat. For a most accurate presentation, place 8 raisins on each cookie to represent the number of eyes a spider has.

3 tablespoons peanut butter

6 round crackers

24 small pretzel sticks

12 raisins

Spread 1½ teaspoons of peanut butter on each cracker. Break the pretzel sticks in half. Push 8 halved sticks into the peanut butter on each cracker, positioning them to make legs. Push 2 raisins into the peanut butter on each cracker to make eyes.

Makes 6 cookies.

PER COOKIE: 86 CAL.; 3G PROT.; 5G FAT; 8G CARB.; 0 CHOL.; 124MG SOD.; 0.7G FIBER.

Fruit Juice Pops

These frozen treats are more delicious than commercial Popsicles and they are full of vitamins—not added sugar.

1 can frozen fruit juice concentrate of choice, thawed

1 to 1½ cans water

Combine the concentrate and water in a bowl. Pour the mixture into 3-ounce paper cups or into Popsicle molds. If using paper cups, let the pops freeze partially, about 1 hour; then insert a Popsicle stick or a blunt toothpick. Freeze until hard, at least 2 hours.

Makes 10 pops.

PER POP: 35 CAL.; 0 PROT.; 0 FAT; 9G CARB.; 0 CHOL.; 5MG SOD.; 0.1G FIBER.

1

Putting It All Together:
The V Diet—Vital, Valid and Vegetarian

The V Diet is vital because it celebrates life. It's valid because it's based on science. It's vegetarian because meatless meals are healthful and delicious.

Whether you're in your first trimester or have tots bent on rearranging your house or teens monopolizing the phone, the V Diet works for everyone. Healthful eating should be a family affair. You are more likely to stick to good eating habits when your family members eat well too. When committed to the vegetarian or near-vegetarian choice, every member in your family will increase his or her odds for a long and healthy life.

Before getting into specifics, here are some guidelines for moms-to-be and children of all ages.

The Five Guidelines of Good Eating

Delight in variety. A healthful vegetarian diet bursts with grains, vegetables, fruits and legumes, and eggs and dairy products if desired. Just choose a variety of foods for balanced nutrition and enjoy.

Eat enough food. A healthful vegetarian diet also provides sufficient calories. A pregnant vegetarian needs about three hundred extra calories daily over her prepregnancy requirements. If you're lactating, you need about five hundred extra calories daily. Once children start eating big-people food, they thrive on three meals a day plus wholesome snacks. As long as they're growing, you can be confident that they're eating enough calories. Don't feed little ones a lot of bulky, high-fiber foods; their tummies may fill up before their caloric needs are met.

Make every bite count. When you choose healthful foods, you will get ample nutrients. A junk-food diet, even if it's vegetarian, is bad news for anyone. Pregnant women who eat poor diets—vegetarian or not—will suffer because their bodies will rob their bones of calcium, for instance, to feed their baby if they shortchange this important mineral. Likewise, children who fill up on nutrient-deficient foods are at greater risk for illness and poor development. Men and nonpregnant women are also smart to make every bite count.

Choose natural foods. That means skipping the newfangled products that line supermarket shelves and loading your cart with foods that are as close as possible to their natural state. Plan on spending lots of time in the produce section of the supermarket or a farm stand, buying foods like whole-wheat flour, dried legumes and grains, and zipping past the aisles with additive-spiked foods whose ingredients you can't pronounce. When you eat natural foods, you will automatically get lots of nutrients and fiber and will decrease your intake of sodium and fat.

Splurge now and then. When you and your children eat a healthful vegetarian diet, it's good to indulge in a favorite but less-than-wholesome food every once in a while. If you become rigid in your eating, you're more likely to slip up and give up. Think balance, not perfection.

A VEGETARIAN EATING PLAN

The Food Guide Pyramid designed by the U.S. Department of Agriculture is an eating guide depicted in a triangle, encouraging Americans to eat more grains, vegetables and fruits. Though it's an improvement over the Four Basic Food Groups, an out-of-date eating guide in which two of the four groups were animal products, the pyramid doesn't meet vegetarians' needs. That's because it overemphasizes meat and dairy products and barely mentions legumes.

Here's a workable plan playing off the pyramid theme. It provides guidelines for healthful eating, ensuring that you and your children will receive ample nutrients and calories. Some of my recommendations are based on a vegetarian food guide published in the *American Journal of Clinical Nutrition*.

Note: Pregnant women should eat the higher number of servings for the milk, yogurt and cheese group or the fortified milk alternatives group. Babies should be breast-fed through the first year if possible; use a commercially prepared infant formula if you don't breast-feed. Young children need only one-fourth to one-half of the serving sizes listed on page 212. Older children and adolescents should eat about the same amount of food as adults. Choose the number of servings based on your caloric needs; the greater your needs, the more daily servings you get.

Food Group	Daily Servings	Serving Size
Breads, grains, cereals (choose 50 percent whole grain)	6 to 11	1 slice bread 1 ounce breakfast cereal ½ cup cooked rice or pasta ½ bagel
Vegetables	3 to 5	½ cup cooked 1 cup raw ¾ cup juice
Fruits	2 to 4	1 medium ½ cup chopped raw or cooked ¼ cup dried ¾ cup juice
Legumes	½ to 2	½ cup cooked ½ cup tofu or tempeh
Milk, yogurt and cheese or milk alternatives fortified with calcium and vitamins D and B_{12}	2 to 3	1 cup milk or yogurt 1½ ounces cheese 1 cup soy milk 1 cup tofu
Eggs	0 to ½	less than 3 yolks a week
Fats, oils, sweets	sparingly except children under two	1 teaspoon butter, margarine or oil 1 ounce nuts or seeds 2 tablespoons nut butter 1 teaspoon sugar, jelly, syrup, etc.

JUST WHEN YOU THOUGHT YOU KNEW IT ALL . . .

Nutrition science is growing up. For instance, just when you've switched your family from butter to margarine to lower their intake of saturated fat, scientists dropped a bomb: Margarine may be worse for health than butter.

Though margarine has minimal saturated fat (11 percent versus the 41 percent in butter), it's teeming with trans fatty acids. Only recently, researchers discovered that trans fatty acids (or "trans fats," for short) can wreak havoc in the body. These fats are formed when vegetable oil is hydrogenated. During hydrogenation, hydrogen atoms are burned into chains of unsaturated fatty acids, causing water and oil to mix. But the heating process produces trans fats, which appear twisted under a microscope.

Not only do trans fats elevate levels of "bad" LDL cholesterol (low-density lipoproteins), but they also cause a drop in "good" HDL cholesterol (high-density lipoproteins). That's bad news: Unhealthful blood cholesterol levels increase your risk for heart disease.

Hydrogenated fats pop up in foods besides margarine. They are in many packaged foods including breads, crackers and cookies. Read package labels. If you see the words "hydrogenated" or "partially hydrogenated" on the label, you know troublesome trans fats lurk inside the box.

FAT MATH

To figure out how much fat you eat, keep track of your food intake for a few days. Then calculate your total number of calories and fat grams, using the following fat-gram counter. Multiply your number of fat grams by 9 because each gram of fat has 9 calories. Then divide this number by your total number of overall calories. The resulting number shows the percent of fat calories in your overall diet. An example: 44 fat grams times 9 equals 396, divided by 2,000 total calories, equals 0.2, or 20 percent.

So should your family switch back to butter? That's a hard question to answer. Butter is highly saturated and contains cholesterol, but margarine has trans fats. And though scientists have a good understanding of the effects of butter on health, they still have a lot to learn about trans fats.

Your best bet: Whenever possible, choose olive, safflower or canola oil in cooking and baking. These fats are very low in saturated fat and contain no trans fats. Most important, keep overall fat consumption to a minimum.

Kids under two years old need a fair amount of fat in their diet for proper growth. But everyone else ought to eat a low-fat diet, with no more than 20 to 25 percent of calories from fat.

That's the latest scientific wisdom. Anticipate updates as researchers learn more. In the science world, nutrition is still a babe . . . but growing up fast. And among the best and most reliable findings: Kids thrive on a healthy vegetarian diet.

2

The Fat-Gram
Counter

Item	Serving Size	Fat Grams
	Breads	
Bagel	1 medium	1
Crackers		
Graham	2 squares	1.3
Saltines	2 crackers	0.6
Croissant	1 medium	12
Doughnut		
Cake	1	8
Yeast	1	14
English muffin	1	1
Pita	1 6-inch round	1
Rice cake	1	0.3
Tortilla		
Corn	1 medium	1.1
Flour	1 large	3.8
Whole-wheat bread	1 slice	0.8

The Fat-Gram Counter

Item	Serving Size	Fat Grams
Cheese		
American		
Reduced calorie	1 ounce	2.2
Regular	1 ounce	8.9
Cheddar		
Reduced calorie	1 ounce	6.5
Regular	1 ounce	9.8
Cottage cheese, 1 percent fat	½ cup	1
Mozzarella, part skim	1 ounce	4.5
Parmesan, grated	1 tablespoon	1.5
Soy cheese	1 ounce	5
Fats		
Butter	1 tablespoon	12.3
Margarine		
Reduced calorie	1 tablespoon	6
Regular	1 tablespoon	12
Oil, all types	1 tablespoon	13.6
Salad dressing		
Regular	1 tablespoon	6 to 8
Low calorie	1 tablespoon	1.5
Fruits		
All	normal portion	less than 1
Grains		
Barley	½ cup cooked	0.8
Bulgur	½ cup cooked	0.5
Cereal		
All-Bran	¾ cup	0.5
Cheerios	1¼ cups	1.8
Granola	⅓ cup	6.5

The Fat-Gram Counter

Item	Serving Size	Fat Grams
Millet	½ cup cooked	0.5
Oats, rolled	½ cup cooked	1.2
Pasta	1 cup cooked	0.8
Rice, brown	½ cup cooked	0.6
Legumes		
All, except for below	½ cup cooked	less than 1
Chickpeas	½ cup cooked	2.2
Soybeans	½ cup cooked	5.1
Tempeh	2 ounces	5.1
Tofu		
Firm	½ cup	11
Soft	½ cup	6
Reduced fat	½ cup	4
Milk, Yogurt and Eggs		
Buttermilk	1 cup	2.2
Eggs		
Boiled	1	5.6
White only	1	0
Evaporated milk		
Skim	½ cup	0.5
Whole	½ cup	10
Milk		
Skim	1 cup	0.4
2 percent	1 cup	4.7
Whole	1 cup	8
Soy milk		
Light	1 cup	2
Regular	1 cup	3.3
Yogurt, low fat	1 cup	2.5
Nuts and Seeds		
Almonds	1 ounce	14.7
Cashews	1 ounce	13.2

The Fat-Gram Counter

Item	Serving Size	Fat Grams
Coconut, dried	1 ounce	18.3
Peanuts	1 ounce	13.9
Peanut butter	1 tablespoon	8.2
Pumpkin seeds	1 ounce	12
Sunflower seeds	1 ounce	14.1

Vegetables

All, except avocado and olives	normal portion	less than 1
Avocado	1 medium	30
Olives, black	4 large	8

Miscellaneous

Cake, without frosting		
Angel food	$\frac{1}{12}$ cake	0.2
Pound	$\frac{1}{12}$ cake	9
Chocolate chips	$\frac{1}{4}$ cup	12.2
Ice milk, vanilla	1 cup	5.6
Popcorn, air-popped	4 cups	0.8
Potato chips	2 ounces	22.4
Pretzels	1 ounce	1
Sherbet	1 cup	0
Sugar, all types	any portion	0

Selected Bibliography

Amato, Paul R., and Partridge, Sonia A. *The New Vegetarians: Promoting Health and Protecting Life*. New York: Plenum Press, 1989.

Barnard, Neil. *Food for Life: How the New Four Food Groups Can Save Your Life*. New York: Crown Publishers, 1993.

Brody, Jane. *Jane Brody's Nutrition Book*. New York: Bantam Books, 1987.

Campbell, T. Colin, et al. *Diet, Lifestyle and Mortality in China: A Study of the Characteristics of 65 Counties*. Oxford University Press, Cornell University Press, and the China People's Medical Publishing House, 1990.

Child Nutrition Program Operations Study: Second Year Report. Office of Analysis and Evaluation, Food and Nutrition Service, U.S. Department of Agriculture, FNS 53–3198–7–32, June 1992.

Committee on Dietary Allowances, Food and Nutrition Board, National Research Council. *Recommended Dietary Allowance*, 10th ed. Washington, D.C.: National Academy Press, 1989.

Diamond, Harvey, and Diamond, Marilyn. *Fit for Life*. New York: Warner Books, 1985.

Eisenberg, Arlene, Murkoff, Heidi E., and Hathaway, Sandee E. *What to Expect When You're Expecting*. New York: Workman Publishing Co., 1991.

Erdman, John, Jr. "Control of Serum Lipids with Soy Protein." *New England Journal of Medicine* 333 (5):313–15 (1995).

Erick, Miriam. *No More Morning Sickness*. New York: Plume, 1993.

Faber, Adele, and Mazlish, Elaine. *How to Talk So Kids Will Listen & Listen So Kids Will Talk*. New York: Avon Books, 1980.

"Fast Facts." *Vegetarian Times*, March 1994.

Gussow, Joan Dye. *Chicken Little, Tomato Sauce and Agriculture*. New York: Bootstrap Press, 1992.

———. "Ecology and Vegetarian Considerations: Does Environmental Responsibility Demand the Elimination of Livestock?" *American Journal of Clinical Nutrition* 59 (suppl.): 1110S–16S (1994).

Haddad, Ella H. "Development of a Vegetarian Food Guide." *American Journal of Clinical Nutrition* 59 (suppl.): 1248S–54S (1994).

Havala, Suzanne, and Dwyer, Johanna. "Position of the American Dietetic Association: Vegetarian Diets." *Journal of the American Dietetic Association* 93:1317–19 (1993).

Howe, Ian. *13th Gen: Abort, Retry, Ignore, Fail?* New York: Vintage Books, 1993.

"Is a Burger Worth It?" *Vegetarian Times,* April 1990.

Jacobson, Michael F., and Maxwell, Bruce. *What Are We Feeding Our Kids?* New York: Workman Publishing Co., 1994.

Krizmanic, Judy. *A Teen's Guide to Going Vegetarian.* New York: Viking, 1994.

Lappé, Frances Moore. *Diet for a Small Planet: 10th Anniversary Edition.* New York: Ballantine Books, 1986.

Lewis, Stephen. "An Opinion on the Global Impact of Meat Consumption." *American Journal of Clinical Nutrition* 59 (suppl.) : 1099S–102S (1994).

McDougall, John A., and McDougall, Mary A. *The McDougall Plan.* Piscataway, N.J.: New Century Publishers, 1983.

Messina, Mark, and Messina, Virginia. *The Simple Soybean and Your Health.* Garden City Park, N.Y.: Avery Publishing, 1994.

Modern Nutrition in Health and Disease, 8th ed. Philadelphia: Lea & Febiger, 1994.

Moll, Lucy, and the editors of *Vegetarian Times. Vegetarian Times Complete Cookbook.* New York: Macmillan, 1995.

Newman, Vicky. "Position of the American Dietetic Association: Promotion and Support of Breast-Feeding." *Journal of the American Dietetic Association* 93:467–69 (1993).

Newman, W. P., et al. "Relation of Serum Lipoprotein Levels and Systolic Blood Pressure in Early Adolescence: The Begalusa Heart Study." *New England Journal of Medicine* 314:138 (1986).

O'Connell, J., et al. "Growth of Vegetarian Children: The Farm Study." *Pediatrics* 84:475–80 (1989).

Ornish, Dean. *Dr. Dean Ornish's Program for Reversing Heart Disease.* New York: Random House, 1990.

Pennington, Jean. *Food Values of Portions Commonly Used,* 15th ed. New York: HarperPerennial, 1989.

Phillips, R. L. "Role of Life-Style and Dietary Habits in the Risk of Cancer Among Seventh-Day Adventists." *Cancer Research* 35:3513–22 (1975).

Phillips, R. L., et al. "Mortality Among California Seventh-Day Adventists for Selected Cancer Sites." *Journal of the National Cancer Institute* 65:1097–1107 (1980).

Rifkin, Jeremy. *Beyond Beef: The Rise and Fall of the Cattle Culture.* New York: Dutton, 1992.

Robbins, John. *Diet for a New America.* Walpole, N.H.: Stillpoint, 1987.

Sanders, T. A. B., and Reddy, Sheela. "Vegetarian Diets and Children." *American Journal of Clinical Nutrition* 59 (suppl.): 1176S–81S (1994).

Spock, Benjamin, and Rothenberg, Michael B. *Dr. Spock's Baby and Child Care.* New York: Pocket Books, 1992.

U.S. Department of Agriculture. *USDA's Food Guide: Background and Development.* Publication no. 1514. Human Nutrition Information Service, 1993.

U.S. Department of Health and Human Services. *Surgeon General's Report on Nutrition and Health.* DHHS Publication no. 88–50210, 1988.

U.S. Preventive Services Task Force. "Routine Iron Supplementation During Pregnancy." *Journal of the American Medical Association* 270 (23):2846–54 (1993).

Wilde, Parke. "Putting a Tired Excuse to Rest." *Vegetarian Times,* February 1992.

Wiley, Carol. "Preteens Sprout Up on Vegetarian Diet." *Vegetarian Times,* April 1990.

Willet, Walter C. "Micronutrients and Cancer Risk." *American Journal of Clinical Nutrition* 59 (suppl.): 1162S–65S (1994).

About the Author

Lucy Moll, the author of the *Vegetarian Times Complete Cookbook*, specializes in writing about food and nutrition. Her passion is health: body, mind and spirit. A ten-year vegetarian and the former executive editor of *Vegetarian Times* magazine, Moll has contributed to *New Woman, Mademoiselle, Health* and other magazines. She lives with her family in Glen Ellyn, Illinois.